VITRECTOMY

Edited by **Zongming Song**

Vitrectomy
Edited by Zongming Song

Published by InTech
Janeza Trdine 9, 51000 Rijeka, Croatia

Notice
Statements and opinions expressed in the chapters are these of the individual contributors and not necessarily those of the editors or publisher. No responsibility is accepted for the accuracy of information contained in the published chapters. The publisher assumes no responsibility for any damage or injury to persons or property arising out of the use of any materials, instructions, methods or ideas contained in the book.

Publishing Process Manager Dejan Grgur

Technical Editor Teodora Smiljanic

Cover Designer InTech Design Team

Additional hard copies can be obtained from orders@intechopen.com

Vitrectomy, Edited by Zongming Song
p. cm.
ISBN 978-953-51-0546-6

For EU product safety concerns:
IN TECH d.o.o., Prolaz Marije Krucifikse Kozulić 3, 51000 Rijeka, Croatia,
info@intechopen.com or visit our website at intechopen.com.

Meet the editor

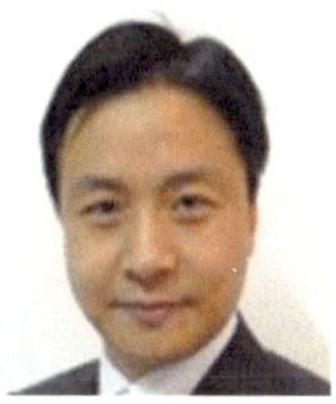

Dr Zongming Song is a Professor of ophthalmology and optometry at Wenzhou Medical College, Adjunct Professor at State University of New York, and Vice Director of Surgical Retina Department, Affiliated Eye Hospital of Wenzhou Medical College. He is also an editorial member of the Chinese Journal of Ocular Fundus Diseases, and reviewer in Retina. Dr Song received his PhD from the Fourth Military Medical University, China in 2001. He specializes in 23/25-gauge minimal invasive vitrectomy for complicated retinal detachment, ocular trauma, diabetic retinopathy and other vitreoretinal diseases. He has more than 4,000 outpatients and annually performs more than 800 operations. He has published over 50 academic papers in top international and Chinese journals such as Ophthalmology, Retina, etc. Dr Song participated in the translation of the book Retina and has given more than 40 academic lectures at international and domestic ophthalmologic annual conferences. He also provides annual Micro-Incision Vitrectomy Surgery training for retinal surgeons nation-wide since 2008.

Contents

Preface IX

Chapter 1 **Vitrectomy in Endophthalmitis 1**
Kapil Bhatia, Avinash Pathengay and Manav Khera

Chapter 2 **Vitrectomy in Open Globe Injuries 17**
Touka Banaee

Chapter 3 **Retinotomy/Retinectomy 39**
Touka Banaee

Chapter 4 **Small Gauge Pars Plana Vitrectomy 55**
Rupan Trikha, Nicole Beharry and David G. Telander

Chapter 5 **Postoperative Tamponade and Positioning Restrictions After Macular Hole Surgery 79**
Yuhei Hasegawa, Yasutaka Mochizuki and Yasuaki Hata

Chapter 6 **Macular Edema Surgical Treatment 89**
Jin Ma

Preface

Since the 1970s, vitrectomy techniques and ophthalmologic tamponade that has been developed and widely applied clinically have greatly improved the treatment for posterior segment oculopathy.

Along with the vitrectomy techniques and equipment updates, the surgical extent and indication are expanding rapidly. Such as from the cornea to subretina; from just posterior segment surgery to combined anterior and posterior segment surgery; from cataract surgery complications, intraocular foreign body removal, endophthalmitis, diabetic retinopathy, complicated retinal detachment, to maculopathy. All novel techniques are based on previous experience that could help new surgeons to avoid mistakes and ensure better service for the patients. There is an abundance of publications about vitreoretinal surgery recently, but the need to introduce the latest advances in the world is still urgent. Therefore, I accepted Mr. Dejan Grgur's invitation to edit this book. The authors in this book are experienced surgeons and researchers who took advantage of new techniques and have extensive academic influence. They have summarized and shared precious experience in this book, which we cannot find in other publications, and this is one of the traits in this book. The book is divided into 6 chapters and I believe many of them have special features we can learn from. The authors have not only shared their experience but also introduced the latest techniques in the world. Since different writers have provided the content of this book, the writing style may be characteristic. Thus, we unify the professional terms and respect their own styles. There are some overlaps among chapters but we have kept these parts to benefit from different authors' views and experiences for discussion.

The goal of this book is to help young surgeons learn about treatment and surgical techniques, and share experience with senior doctors. Due to limitations in our own knowledge, I hope the readers will hold a critical attitude and give comments in order to improve the future editions.

Zongming Song, MD
Professor of Ophthalmology, Adjunct Professor, State University of New York
USA
Vice Director, Surgical Retina Department,
Affiliated Eye Hospital of Wenzhou Medical College
China

1

Vitrectomy in Endophthalmitis

Kapil Bhatia, Avinash Pathengay and Manav Khera
Retina Vitreous Services, L.V. Prasad Eye Institute,
GMR Varalakshmi Campus, Visakhapatnam
India

1. Introduction

Endophthalmitis is a severe, purulent intraocular inflammation of the intraocular cavities (i.e. the aqueous or vitreous humor) usually caused by infection. Endophthalmitis can be exogenous or endogenous.

Exogenous is caused by trauma or surgery (most commonly cataract extraction).

Approximately 70 percent of cases occur as a direct complication of intraocular surgery. Such post-operative endophthalmitis may be acute (presenting within 6 weeks of surgery) or chronic. Incidence of acute endophthalmitis following cataract extraction have been reported between 0.072% and 0.13% in various studies.[1-4] The most common infecting organisms following cataract extraction are the coagulase-negative *Staphylococcus spp.*, especially S. *epidermidis*.[5,6]

Endogenous (metastatic) endophthalmitis is caused by organisms reaching the eye via blood stream. In endogenous endophthalmitis, blood-borne organisms permeate the blood-ocular barrier either by direct invasion (e.g. septic emboli) or by changes in vascular endothelium caused by substrates released during infection. Destruction of intraocular tissues may be due to direct invasion by the organism and/or from inflammatory mediators of the immune response. It is seen in patients in whom body immunity is compromised e.g. chronic alcoholics, HIV patients, malignancy, renal transplant patients.

The management of endophthalmitis revolves around intense medical treatment and surgical intervention, with salvaging the eye and vision as primary aim (Table 1). Diagnosis and intensive treatment at the earliest possible time is essential. The timing is controversial and needs surgeon's judgment regarding immediate or delayed surgical intervention taking into account the risk and benefit to the patient (Table 2).

2. Endophthalmitis Vitrectomy Study (EVS)

Before the EVS, there were widely divergent opinions regarding the role of vitrectomy in endophthalmitis management, ranging from vitrectomy for all endophthalmitis cases to the use of vitrectomy for only the most severe cases with greater inflammation, worse visual acuity, and more rapid onset. Great strides were made for post cataract endophthalmitis with the execution of the prospective Endophthalmitis Vitrectomy Study (EVS) in the 1990s

Aim's of management
• Kill the organism; • Remove the inflammatory debris from the vitreous cavity • Block the inflammatory cascade and its effects on the retina • Treat the complications of the infection

Table 1. Summarizes the aims of management in endophthalmitis.

Immediate vitrectomy:	Delayed vitrectomy:
1. Obtains early sample for vitreous culture and to start specific treatment.	1. Easier to operate on a non inflamed eye
2. Clears ocular media to assess disease severity and treatment response.	2. Tissue is less friable
3. Removes toxic products/ vitreous scaffold for the formation of scar tissue as also the vitreous membranes which could lead to tractional retinal detachment.	3. Visualization is better
4. Reduces bacterial load	
5. Intravitreal antibiotics at the end of procedure.	
6. Increases the antibiotics concentration in the eye. It also facilitates better diffusion and penetration of antibiotics as they are delivered directly to the infected site during vitrectomy.	
7. Increases retinal oxygenization	
8. Reduces the incidence and severity of retinal, especially macular, complications.	

Table 2. Denotes the advantages of performing immediate vitrectomy over delayed vitrectomy in endophthalmitis.

to lay the guidelines for the timings of vitrectomy.[7] The EVS evaluated the role of immediate pars plana vitrectomy versus intraocular antibiotic injection (TAP) and systemic antibiotics in the treatment of acute postoperative endophthalmitis. Acute post-operative endophthalmitis (presenting within 6 weeks) and secondary IOL implantation patients who were having an initial visual acuity between 20/50 and light perception, and had a view sufficient to perform a vitrectomy were included in the study. 420 patients were randomized to immediate initial TAP or vitrectomy. There was no difference in final visual outcomes in patients who underwent initial TAP or vitrectomy if presenting visual acuity was better than light perception. However, in patients presenting with light perception vision, those who underwent initial vitrectomy were 3 times more likely to achieve 20/40 vision or better, twice as likely to maintain 20/100 vision or better, and had a nearly 50% reduction in the risk of severe visual loss (< 5/200), compared to patients who underwent TAP. No long-term difference occurred in media clarity between the treatment groups.

3. Pitfalls of EVS

Although EVS study did give us first insight and guidelines, but there were various pitfalls present in the study itself. Since the EVS specifically excluded patients with postoperative endophthalmitis who underwent any procedure other than cataract surgery, results cannot be generalized to every endophthalmitis. In patients with conjunctival filtering bleb-associated endophthalmitis, earlier vitrectomy is preferred because of more profound inflammation and the increased probability of more virulent organisms. Further traumatic endophthalmitis (especially associated with intraocular foreign body) presents with intense inflammation and if vitrectomy is not done early, it can lead to loss of the eye. Chronic post-operative endophthalmitis (caused by P.*acne* or fungus) has been associated with high rates of persistent inflammation. Vitrectomy with special attention to either partial or total capsular bag excision with or without IOL removal has been reported effective in eradicating inflammation as compared to TAP alone. Further newer generations systemic antibiotics can achieve good concentration inside the eye, and help in reducing the infection and achieving having good outcome. Technological advancements in vitreoretinal surgery since EVS have minimized the risks associated with vitrectomy favoring the initial use of vitrectomy in less severe cases also.

4. Procedure

Before starting surgical intervention, necessary instruments and drugs should be ready. (Table 3)

• **Instruments:**	• **Disposables:**	• **Medication:**
- Eye speculum	- Surgical drape	- 0.5% Bupivacaine
- Forceps	- Sterile surgical gloves	- 2% lidocaine
- Irrigation cannula	- 10% povidone iodine swabs	- 150 IE Hyaluronidase
- Corneo-scleral scissors	- 5% povidone iodine solution	- 0.1 cc Cetazidime (22.5 mg/ml)
- Vitrectome hand piece and unit	- Three plastic cups	- 0.1 cc Vancomycin (10 mg/ml)
- Barraquer forceps	- One syringe (6.0 cc)	- 0.1 cc Dexamethasone (4 mg/ml)
	- Four syringes (1.0 cc)	
	- Cotton tip applicators	
	- Three 30-gauge needles	
	- Three sterile caps for syringes	
	- 4×4-cm sterile cotton pads	
	- 23-gauge microvitreoretinal blade	
	- Eye pad and tape	

Table 3. Signifies equipment required for the management of endophthalmitis

5. Vitreous tap

This procedure is preferably done under peribulbar anaesthesia using 2% lignocaine and/or 0.5% bupivacaine. As with routine surgery, eye has to be prepared using povidone-iodine scrub followed by sterile drape. Vitreous tap can be done either with a needle attached to a syringe or using the vitreous cutter.

A 5 cc syringe and small gauge needle (23-26G) is preferred for the aspiration. A 23 gauge butterfly needle can also be used for this purpose. The needle is inserted approximately 3-4mm (3mm for aphakic, 3.5mm for pseudophakic and 4 mm for phakic patients) from the limbus into the mid vitreous cavity. Gentle aspiration is applied and 0.2-0.3 ml of fluid is aspirated. If vitreous is not aspirated, the needle tip can be carefully moved in an attempt to locate a pocket of liquid vitreous. If after several attempts a vitreous specimen cannot be obtained the procedure should be terminated as suction can lead to iatrogenic retinal tears formation and subsequent retinal detachment.In such kind of cases one could use vitreous cutter to tap the vitreous. Intraocular antibiotics can be injected at the same sitting. Vancomycin (1mg in 0.1 ml), and ceftazidime (2.25 mg in 0.1ml) are the preferred drugs initially till the final microbiology report is available. Doses of various intravitreal antibiotic chart should be prepared and should be pasted in operation theatre as doses are confusing, and slight mistake in making can lead to adverse events (e.g. toxicity). Common intravitreal antibiotics doses and their mechanism of action have been described in (Table 4).

6. Vitrectomy

The surgical technique of vitrectomy is similar to the standard three-port vitrectomy with few exceptions. Securing the infusion cannula correctly is very important and its visualization through an inflammed choroid and hazy media can be a difficult thing. A longer infusion cannula (6-mm cannula), is generally recommended in these situations. If cannula is still not visible then a good alternative is to use the hand held infusion cannula and clear vitreous exudates with the cutter till the regular cannula is visible through the pupil. If the epithelium is edematous, its removal may be necessary. Scraping the epithelium can increases the visibility and thus increases the success rate of the surgery. If the stroma also has significant edema, pressing a dry sponge against it, or using topical high-concentration glucose may increase visibility. The anterior chamber often contains hypopyon and exudative membrane which interferes with adequate visualization. In pseudophakic patients a 26-gauge instrument, such as, a hypodermic needle could be introduced through the limbus to clear the hypopyon and any inflammatory membrane without explantation of the IOL or anterior chamber maintainer can be used and inflammatory material over IOL can be aspirated to make visualization better. Vitreous aspirate should be the first step of the surgery before starting the infusion to get an undiluted sample for culture. Vitreous sample is collected by short tubing attached to the suction port of the vitrectomy probe. The suction is operated manually by syringe attached to the tubing. Infusion fluid bottle should be at a low height. Care should be taken not to cause too much hypotony while taking vitreous aspirate and as soon as biopsy is obtained, infusion should be switched on, and suction should be very slow so as not to cause any inadvertent traction leading to break formation. The aim of vitrectomy in endophthalmitis is

ANTIBIOTICS	DOSE	MECHANISM OF ACTION
Amikacin	0.4mg/0.1ml	Inhibit protein synthesis by binding to the 30S rRNA molecule of the bacterial ribosome
Kanamycin	0.5mg/0.1ml	Inhibit protein synthesis by binding to the 30S rRNA molecule of the bacterial ribosome
Tobramycin	0.4mg/0.1ml	Inhibit protein synthesis by binding to the 30S rRNA molecule of the bacterial ribosome
Vancomycin	1.0mg/o.1ml	Inhibit protein synthesis by binding to the 30S rRNA molecule of the bacterial ribosome
Ampicillin	5.omg/0.1ml	Inhibition of bacterial cell wall synthesis by preventing the cross linking of peptides on the mucosaccharide chains
Carbenicillin	2.0mg/0.1ml	Inhibition of bacterial cell wall synthesis by preventing the cross linking of peptides on the mucosaccharide chains
Methicillin	2.0mg/0.1ml	Inhibition of bacterial cell wall synthesis by preventing the cross linking of peptides on the mucosaccharide chains
Erythromycin	0.5mg/0.1ml	Inhibit protein synthesis by binding to the 23S rRNA molecule (in the 50S subunit) of the bacterial ribosome blocking the exit of the growing peptide chain
Gentamicin	0.2mg/0.1ml	Inhibit protein synthesis by binding to the 30S rRNA molecule of the bacterial ribosome
Cefazoline	2.0mg/0.1ml	Inhibition of bacterial cell wall synthesis by preventing the cross linking of peptides on the mucosaccharide chains
Ceftazidime	2.25mg/0.1ml	Inhibition of bacterial cell wall synthesis by preventing the cross linking of peptides on the mucosaccharide chains
Imipenum	0.05mg/0.1ml	Inhibition of synthesis of the peptidoglycan layer of bacterial cell walls
Tazobactum	2.25mg/0.1ml	Inhibition of bacterial cell wall synthesis
ANTIFUNGALS		
Amphotericin B	0.5mg/0.1ml	Associates with ergosterol forming a transmembrane channel that leads to monovalent ion (K^+, Na^+, H^+ and Cl^-) leakage
Voriconazole	0.05mg/0.1ml	Inhibition of fungal-cytochrome P-450-mediated 14 alpha- lanosterol demethylation, leading to an accumulation of 14 alpha-methyl sterols which results in loss of ergosterol in the cell wall

Table 4. Summarizes the dose of intravitreal antimicrobial agents and mechanism of actions of these drugs used in the management of endophthalmitis.

only to perform a "core" vitrectomy. There should be minimal traction on the inflamed and friable retina. To avoid unnecessary traction, vitrectomy should be performed with low suction and high cut rate. PVD (posterior vitreous detachment) induction should be avoided as it can lead to traction and can lead to break formation leading to rhegmatogenous retinal detachment. IOL explantation is not necessary in all the cases of pseudophakic endophthalmitis.[8, 9] Explantation of the IOL is mostly necessary in fungal endophthalmitis and in *P. acnes* endophthalmitis, however one should try to preserve IOL as far as possible and perform a generous capsulotomy, either to retain or exchange the IOL and to inject intraocular antibiotic near the remaining part of the capsular bag.[10] IOL explantation should be reserved as a last option.

7. Endophthalmitis in phakic patients

The above mentioned procedure holds good if patients is aphakic or having intraocular lens (IOL) implanted. Endophthalmitis in phakic patients presents with difficult situation (e.g. traumatic or endogenous endophthalmitis). Lens can be clear with major involvement of posterior segment or lens can be involved (lens abscess). Preserving the lens has the advantage of preserving the natural lens, and it increases the half-life of intraocular antibiotics.[32] In a study by Huang et al, authors were able to control the infections in all the eyes (12 eyes) without removing the natural lens.[33] Six of 12 eyes achieved 20/80 or better visual acuity with an average follow-up time of 13 months. Six of eight eyes treated with pars plana vitrectomy and intraocular antibiotic injection achieved this level of visual acuity in contrast to none of four eyes treated with only intraocular antibiotic injection. [33] If infection is severe and media is hazy because of lens, one should not be hesitant to remove lens, so as to have better visualization to complete vitrectomy and achieve good visual outcome. IOL placement can be done as a secondary procedure at later date once infection is well controlled. However one should try to preserve lens as far as possible.

8. Extent of vitrectomy

There is a variable consensus on the extent of the vitrectomy. According to the EVS study, only core vitrectomy should be done and posterior vitreous detachment (PVD) should be avoided as far as possible, as retina is inflammed and friable and there are high chances of retinal break formation. Core vitrectomy comprises the removal of anterior and central vitreous first, followed by posterior central vitreous. No attempt is made to enter vitreous base. No posterior hyaloid cleaning is done. Core vitrectomy is only done in central area and peripheral vitrectomy should be avoided. End point of vitrectomy is either when red glow is visible or disc with 1st order vessels are visible. Intravitreal antibiotics are injected at the end of the procedure. As opposed to conservative vitrectomy (recommended by EVS and followed mostly), induction of PVD and little more aggressive vitrectomy was advocated in complete and early vitrectomy for endophthalmitis (CEVE).[11] Authors in their series of 47 consecutive postoperative endophthalmitis patients found statistically significantly better anatomical and functional results with CEVE than in either management arm in the EVS. The authors attribute this improvement to vitrectomy being early and complete, and to its being the primary line of treatment, rather than being applied as a last resort.[11] According to author PVD induction should only be done at posterior pole over non-necrotic area. PVD should not be attempted aggressively or should not be extended beyond equator, as there are high chances of teat formation with subsequent retinal detachment. Further posterior exudates over the surface of retina can be aspirated by soft tip flute needle. PVD induction will have direct access of antibiotics to retinal surfaces and removes posterior vitreous scaffold for infection, leading to early recovery.

During vitrectomy surgeon should be extremely careful to cut anything as there are several vitreous layers and membranes can be present and sometimes it is very difficult to differentiate them from the retina esp. when there are streaks of blood among the layers, giving the appearance of a detached retina. Further retina can become necrotic in endophthalmitis leading to white avascular appearance simulating vitreous layers, and even on cutting it does not bleed. A less experienced or careful surgeon may remove large area of the retina before realizing it. To avoid this complication, surgeon should not cut any membrane without visualization. Vitrectomy should be started from behind the lens and then slowly one should advance towards the retina. If there is doubt regarding the structures, its better to do vitrectomy in nasal quadrant to avoid inadvertent injury to the fovea. If still it is not possible to differentiate the retina from the vitreous, its better to do very minimal vitrectomy and plan repeat surgery later once the media clarity improves a little, rather than doing more harm to the patient. Many a time's visibility is the major concern in performing vitrectomy and extent of vitrectomy depends entirely upon the visualization.. There are several options:

- Vitrectomy may be performed in a limited fashion, ("Proportional pars plana vitrectomy"[PPPV], a term coined by R. Morris).[12] It is always better to perform vitreous tap with limited core vitrectomy rather than inflicting severe damage because of poor visualization.
- A temporary keratoprosthesis (TKP) can be placed followed by implantation of donor cornea at the conclusion of surgery. If no donor cornea is available, even the original corneal button may be temporarily reused.
- An endoscope may be utilized. But considerable experience is required on surgeon's part and availability is also the major problem.

Surgical procedure mentioned above cannot be applied to all the cases of endophthalmitis, as, post-traumatic and bleb related endophthalmitis are very difficult to manage and chronic endophthalmitis presents a very different clinical challenge to the clinician. So surgical modifications have to be adopted based on clinical presentation.

9. Acute-onset postoperative endophthalmitis

Acute postoperative endophthalmitis usually presents within 6 weeks of the surgery. It can present after any intraocular surgery, but it is most common after cataract surgery. Most common organism implicated is coagulase-negative staphylococci, but *Staphylococcus aureus*, the *Streptococcus* species, and gram-negative organisms can also cause postoperative endophthalmitis. As EVS study was done for post-operative endophthalmitis, so the results can be safely followed here. Early cases of endophthalmitis can be treated with vitreous TAP along with intravitreal antibiotics, but for severe cases PPV is the treatment of choice (figure 1 a,b). Presenting visual acuity was the single most important factor in EVS predicting the

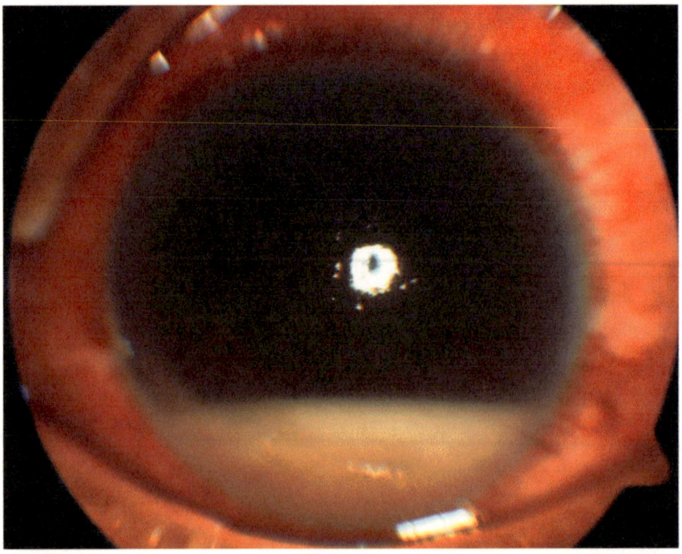

a.

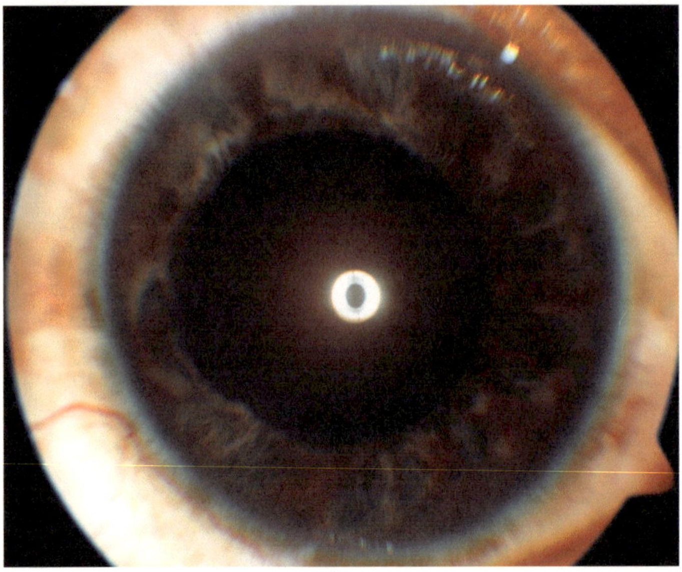

b.

Fig. 1. Photographs of the left eye of 55 yr male presenting with acute endophthalmitis of bacterial origin a. Presenting VA: HM, IOP: 18 mmHg. Treatment: pars plana vitrectomy with intravitreal Vancomycin, Ceftazidime, and Dexamethasone. b. At 3 months VA:20/40, IOP:14 mmHg.

final visual acuity. In EVS, 23% of patients with light perception acuity achieved 20/40 or better final acuity, compared with 64% of patients who had hand motions or better acuity. This data signifies the need for early treatment before severe visual loss happens (regardless whether TAP or vitrectomy is done). Once patient presents with severe visual loss, vitrectomy has better visual outcome and is the treatment of choice. Role of intravitreal steroid is controversial in these cases. Since 90% of these cases are caused by bacteria, so early steroid administration reduces the inflammation and increases the chances of visual recovery (figure 2 a,b). In a prospective randomized clinical trial of 63 bacterial endophthalmitis cases Das et al, found that intravitreal dexamethasone reduces inflammation scores early in the course of treatment but had no independent influence on the final visual outcome.[13] So the role of steroids is still controversial.

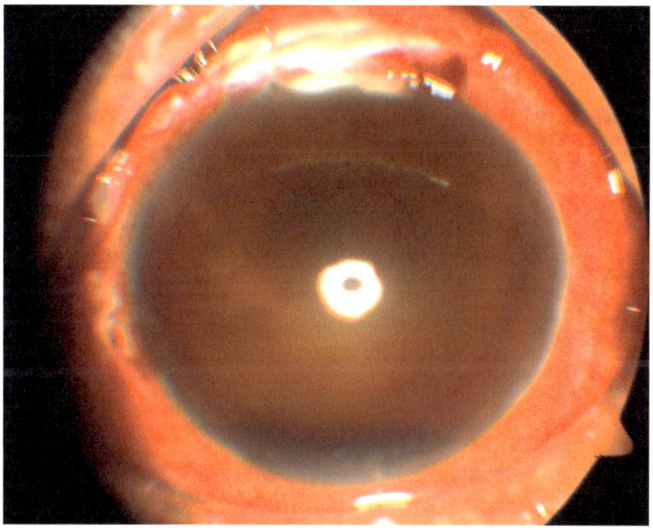

a.

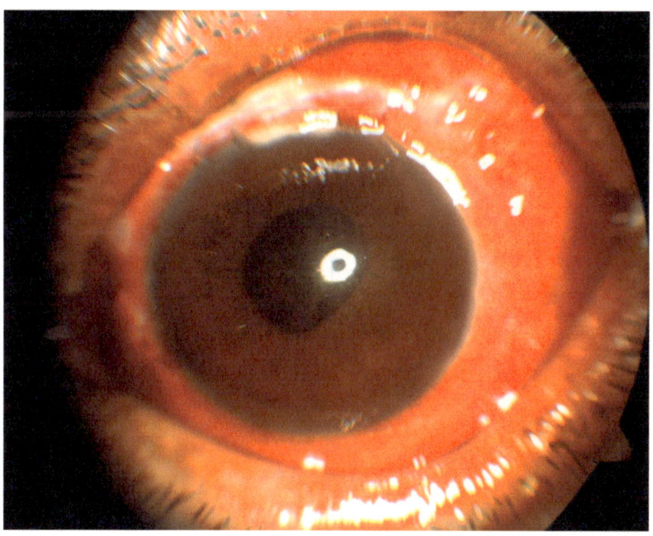

b.

Fig. 2. Photographs of the eye of 40 yr male presenting with acute postoperative endophthalmitis with scleral tunnel infiltrate (culture negative) a. Presenting VA: HM. Treatment: pars plana vitrectomy with intravitreal Vancomycin, Ceftazidime, Dexamethasone, tunnel resuturing. Patient received 4 IOAB + dexamethasone injections after initial PPV. b. At 3 months VA:20/60.

10. Delayed-onset or chronic postoperative endophthalmitis

Endophthalmitis patients presenting after 6 weeks (months to year), are included in chronic endophthalmitis. They present not only with diagnostic challenge, but their management is vastly different from acute onset counterpart. *Propionibacterium acnes,* a gram-positive, anaerobic rod, is the most common organism causing chronic endophthalmitis. Characteristic feature of P.acne endophthalmitis is whitish capsular plaque (organisms mixed with residual lens cortex), which can be mistaken for posterior capsular opacification. Since organisms are residing inside capsular bag, simple vitrectomy with intravitreal antibiotics generally leads to inferior result with recurrence of infection. A pars plana vitrectomy and a central capsulectomy together with intravitreal antibiotics (vancomycin is the drug of choice) is generally recommended as the first line management.[14-16] Vancomycin is injected into capsular bag at the end of the procedure. If infection is still not controlled; IOL removal along with complete bag removal is the treatment of choice. In clinically suspected fungal infections (2nd most common cause of chronic endophthalmitis) characterized by fluffy vitreous infiltrates with white snow ball like opacities, immediate injection of antifungal agents (intravitreal amphotericin B 5 μg or voriconazole 100 ug), is recommended after vitrectomy. If still infection is not controlled, total capsulectomy and IOL removal should be considered.[17, 18]

11. Posttraumatic endophthalmitis

In contrast to acute postoperative endophthalmitis, posttraumatic endophthalmitis carries worse prognosis (high severity of infection, polymicrobial etiology, associated pathologies e.g. IOFB, RD). *Bacillus* species, most commonly *B. cereus,* is the most common organism (cultured positivity 28% to 46%).[19, 20] Endophthalmitis caused by *Bacillus* species is progressive, and generally carries a poor visual prognosis, even after immediate vitrectomy.[21-23] Traumatic endophthalmitis esp. associated with retained intraocular foreign body (IOFB) carries the worst prognosis. In one study 3.5% patients with retained foreign bodies developed endophthalmitis when the primary surgical repair was accomplished within 24 hours of the injury compared with 13.4% patients in whom the primary surgical repair was delayed more than 24 hours.[24] Further only 40.9% culture-positive cases achieved 20/400 or better visual acuity necessitating the need for early vitrectomy and removal of IOFB. If retinal break or retinal detachment is also present, complete vitrectomy with endolaser of break with silicone oil injection is warranted to achieve good anatomical outcome.

12. Endogenous endophthalmitis

It is commonly seen in patients in whom body immunity is compromised e.g. chronic alcoholics, HIV patients, malignancy, renal transplant patients. Most common organisms implicated are bacteria or fungus (candida, aspergillus). The timing of and necessity for vitrectomy remains unclear in endogenous as compared with postoperative endophthalmitis. Vitrectomy will be more useful in posterior diffuse disease and severe disease (figure 3 a,b). In cases of fungal endophthalmitis, vitrectomy provides a good specimen for microbiology and effectively reduces the number of organisms. It is also crucial to consider the overall status of these individuals, many of whom will be desperately

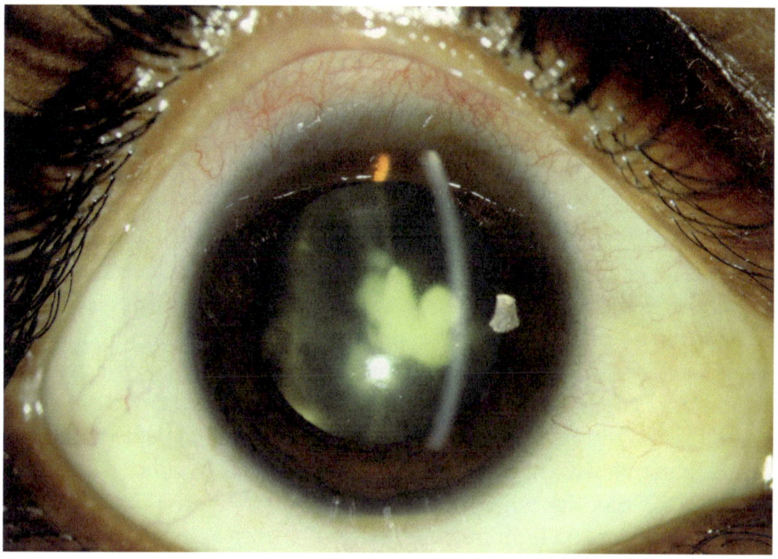

a.

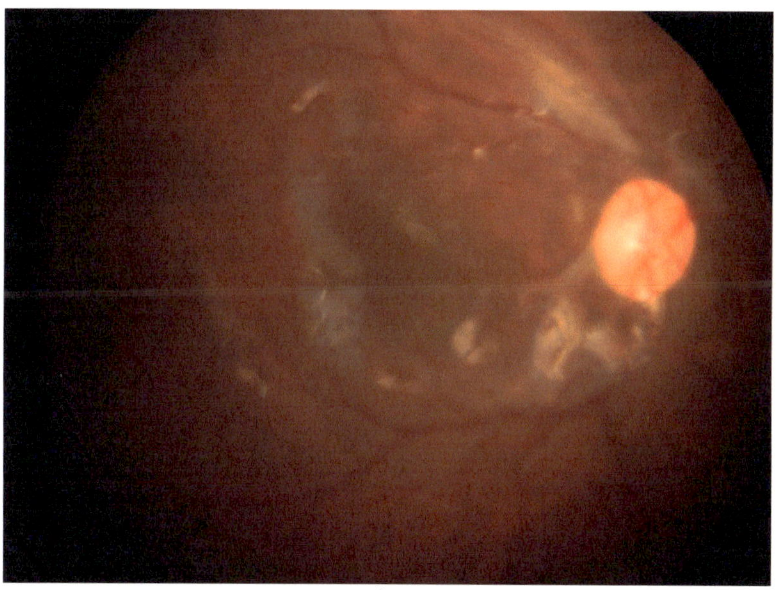

b.

Fig. 3. Photographs of the right eye of 22 yr male presenting with acute endogenous endophthalmitis (gram negative bacilli) a. Presenting VA: PL PR ACCURATE. Treatment: pars plana vitrectomy with intravitreal Vancomycin, Ceftazidime, and Dexamethasone. Patient developed RD for which PPV+EL+SIO was done. b. At 3 months VA:20/30.

ill from systemic sepsis and anesthesia risk for surgery is very high. Despite aggressive antimicrobial therapy, most patients with endogenous endophthalmitis have a poor outcome. In a study from Singapore over a 4-year period, 17 of 32 affected eyes ended up with no light perception even after early surgical intervention.[25]

13. Bleb associated endophthalmitis

The organisms frequently involved in this type of endophthalmitis include streptococcal species and *Haemophilus influenzae.* These organisms liberate potent toxins and tissue damaging enzymes that may contribute to virulence of intraocular infection and associated intraocular inflammation. The treatment of infections with such organisms poses serious problems. Even if the intraocular spaces are sterilised with appropriate antibiotics, a significant amount of bacterial debris and potentially toxic products remain to account for treatment failure. Hence pars plana vitrectomy and intraocular antibiotics are considered as the first line of management. Inspite of early and aggressive approach, visual outcome is not satisfactory. Song et al in their series of post bleb related endophthalmitis found that patients who underwent prompt pars plana vitrectomy (PPV)generally had a worse final visual outcome when compared with the tap/inject group.[26] Busbee et al however found contrasting results with regard to treatment modality in the 68 patients with bleb associated endophthalmitis. Patients who underwent PPV had a greater likelihood of retaining 20/100 vision or better at 12 months when compared with tap/inject (33% vs 13%, P = 0.09). Significantly higher rates of no light perception (NLP) vision were also seen in patients with a positive culture or who underwent tap/inject as primary treatment indicating early need for the vitrectomy.[27] Dexamethasone can be used as along with antibiotics, as it will reduce the inflammatory damage induced by toxins thereby limiting the visual loss. However final visual acuity was same in dexamethasone receiving endophthalmitis group as well as in other group not receiving the drug as reported in literature.[13, 27]

A brief summarization regarding the treatment and outcome of these types of endophthalmitis is given below (Table 5).

	Acute Postop. Endophthalmitis	Delayed/Chronic Postop. Endophthalmitis	Bleb Associated Endophthalmitis	Endogenous Endophthalmitis	Traumatic Endophthalmitis
Causative organism	Coagulase negative *Staphylococci*	*P.Acne*, Fungi, *Staphylococcus epidermidis*	*Streptococcus, Hemophilus*	Bacteria, Fungi	*Bacilli*, Fungi, Mixed
Treatment of choice	PPV/TAP+IOAB	PPV ± IOL explantation ± Capsular bag removal + IOAB	PPV + IOAB	PPV/TAP + IOAB	PPV+IOAB ± additional procedure
Indications of vitrectomy	Severe infection, presenting vision PL±, worsening clinical picture	Recurrent episodes, white capsular plaque, fungal etiology	Mostly all cases	Severe infection, presenting vision PL±, worsening clinical picture	Mostly preferred esp. associated with IOFB, suspected fungal etiology
Prognosis	Depends on initial visual Acuity, organism virulence	Variable	Poor	Poor	Poor

Table 5. Summarization of treatment option and prognosis of various types of endophthalmitis

14. Complications

Vitrectomy procedure for endophthalmitis carries high complication rates because of several reasons. Various complications that commonly occur during vitrectomy are:

1. **Retinal break**: Breaks can occur as a normal complication, as a direct injury from an intravitreal instrument, or as a result of aggressive vitrectomy to induce PVD. The breaks can be surrounded with laser or silicone oil may be used.
2. **Retinal Detachment**: Retinal detachment can be rhegmatogenous (retinal break, surgical complication), tractional or exudative. Retina is very friable and necrotic in endophthalmitis, so chances of break formation with subsequent retinal detachment are very high.
3. Vitreous hemorrhage
4. Retinal toxicity from antibiotics
5. Phthisis bulbi

In the EVS, major adverse events included retinal detachment in 5%, phthisis in 3%. Compared with TAP, vitrectomy was associated with a slightly lower rate of complications. Retinal detachment and phthisis occurred in 2.7% and 2% of vitrectomy eyes, respectively, compared to 7% and 4% of TAP group. However incidence of late additional surgical procedure did not differ whether vitrectomy was performed or initial procedure was TAP. The incidence of late additional surgical procedures was 27% overall.[31]

15. Role of introcular tamponade

Routine endophthalmitis surgery does not require any tamponade. However tamponade is necessary if any complication happens. Retinal with subsequent retinal detachment requires long term tamponade. Silicone oil can be used in cases where retinal break formation or retinal detachment has occurred. Not only it provides a long term tamponade, but it also retards the infectious process, as bacteria do not grow in silicone oil. However one should try to remove as much vitreous possible before injecting oil. Further doses of intravitreal injections has to be reduced (in general half the normal dosage), as oil prolongs their half-life and if normal doses are injected there are high chances of retinal toxicity.

Finally vitrectomy for endophthalmitis can also be done using suturless (23 or 25 gauge) system. There appears to be a trend toward the use of smaller gauge vitrectomy systems. Possible advantages include shorter operating time, reduced post operative inflammation from sutures in an already inflamed eye, reduced incidence of post operative retinal tears and detachments.[28] Hilton et al; have evaluated office based suturless pars plana vitrectomy for various diseases including endophthalmitis with good success.[29]

Tan et al, reviewed the outcomes of 23G vitrectomy in patients with postoperative endophthalmitis and found it to be a useful technique. There was no case of postoperative hypotony or wound leak.[30]

In summary vitrectomy helps in debulking of vitreous, allowing dispersion of intra-ocular antibiotics and facilitating clearing of the visual pathway. Microbiological diagnosis is best made by culture of vitreous aspirate. Therapeutic vitrectomy is reserved for severe cases, defined as vitreous inflammation severe enough to obstruct view of the posterior pole on indirect ophthalmoscopy, progressive inflammation despite initial antibiotic therapy, and/or cases that have not improved despite initial therapy. The need for additional procedures is a marker of more severe disease and is usually associated with worse visual outcomes. However, management of patients should be individualized and should be based on clinical judgment.

16. References

[1] Aaberg TM Jr, Flynn HW Jr, Schiffman J, Newton J. Nosocomial acute-onset postoperative endophthalmitis survey. A 10-yr review of incidence and outcomes. Ophthalmology. 1998;105:1004–10.

[2] Powe NR, Schein OD, Gieser SC, et al. Synthesis of the literature on visual acuity and complications after cataract extraction with intraocular lens implantation. Arch Ophthalmol. 1994;112:239–52.

[3] Javitt JC, Vitale S, Canner JK, et al. National outcomes of cataract extraction: endophthalmitis after inpatient surgery. Arch Ophthalmol. 1991;109:1085–9.

[4] Kattan HM, Flynn HW Jr, Pflugfelder SC, et al. Nosocomial endophthalmitis survey. Current incidence of infection after intraocular surgery. Ophthalmology. 1991;98:227–38.

[5] Han DP, Wisniewski SR, Wilson LA, et al. Spectrum and susceptibilities of microbiologic isolates in the Endophthalmitis Vitrectomy Study. Am J Ophthalmol. 1996;122:1–17

[6] Kunimoto DY, Das T, Sharma S, et al. Microbiologic spectrum and susceptibility of isolates: part I. Postoperative endophthalmitis. Endophthalmitis Research Group. Am J Ophthalmol. 1999;128:240–2.

[7] Endophthalmitis Vitrectomy Study Group: Results of the Endophthalmitis Vit- rectomy Study: a randomized trial of immediate vitrectomy and of intravenous antibiotics for the treatment of postoperative bacterial endophthalmitis. Arch Ophthalmol 1995;13:1479–1496.

[8] Driebe W, Mandelbaum S, Forster RK. Pseudophakic endophthalmitis: Diagnosis and management. Ophthalmology 1986;93:442-447.

[9] Hopen G, Mondino BJ, Kozy D, et al. Intraocular lenses and experimental bacterial endophthalmitis. Am J Ophthalmol 1982;94:402-407.

[10] Benson WE. Current management of postsurgical endophthalmitis. In:The Year book of Ophthalmology, Laibson PR, ed. Chicago, Year Book Medical Publishers Inc., 1989, pp. 181-184.

[11] Kuhn F, Gini G. Complete and early vitrectomy for endophthalmitis (CEVE) as today's alternative to the Endophthalmitis vitrectomy study. Vitreo retinal surgery: Essentials in ophthalmology. 2007;Chapter 5:53-68.

[12] Morris R, Witherspoon CD, Kuhn F, Bryne JB, Endophthalmitis. In: Roy FH (1995) Masters techniques in ophthalmology. Williams and Wilkins, pp 560–572.

[13] Das T, Jalali S, Gothwal V, et al.: Intravitreal dexamethasone in exogenous bacterial endophthalmitis: result of a prospective randomized study. Br J Ophthalmol 1999;83:1050–5.

[14] Clark WL, Kaiser PK, Flynn HW Jr, et al.: Treatment strategies and visual acuity outcomes in chronic postoperative *P. acnes* endophthalmitis. Ophthalmology 1999;106:1665–70.
[15] Aldave AJ, Stein JD, Deramo VA, et al.: Treatment strategies for postoperative *Propionibacterium acnes* endophthalmitis. Ophthalmology 1999;106:2395–401.
[16] TA: Update on acute and chronic endophthalmitis. Ophthalmology 1999;106:2237–8.
[17] Stern WH, Tamura E, Jacobs RA, et al.: Epidemic postsurgical *Candida parapsilosis* endophthalmitis: clinical findings and management of 15 consecutive cases. Ophthalmology 1985;92:170.
[18] Petit TH, Olson RJ, Foos RY, et al.: Fungal endophthalmitis following intraocular lens implantation. A surgical epidemic. Arch Ophthalmol 1980;98:1025.
[19] Brinton GS, Topping TM, Hyndiuk RA, et al.: Posttraumatic endophthalmitis. Arch Ophthalmol 1984;102:547.
[20] Thompson JT, Parver LM, Enger C, et al.: Endophthalmitis after penetrating ocular injuries with retained intraocular foreign bodies. Ophthalmology 1993;100:1468.
[21] Vahey JB, Flynn HW Jr: Results in the management of *Bacillus* endophthalmitis. Ophthalmic Surg 1991;22:681.
[22] Hemady R, Zaltas M, Paton B, et al.: *Bacillus*-induced endophthalmitis: new series of 10 cases and review of the literature. Br J Ophthalmol 1990;74:26.
[23] Foster RE, Martinez JA, Murray TG, et al.: Useful visual outcomes after treatment of *Bacillus cereus* endophthalmitis. Ophthalmology 1996;103:390–7.
[24] Thompson JT, Parver LM, Enger C, et al.: Endophthalmitis after penetrating ocular injuries with retained intraocular foreign bodies. Ophthalmology 1993;100:1468.
[25] Wong JS, Chan TK, Lee HM, Chee SP. Endogenous bacterial endophthalmitis: an east Asian experience and a reappraisal of a severe ocular affliction. Ophthalmology 2000;107:1483-91.
[26] Song A, Scott IU, Flynn HWJr, et al.: Delayed-onset bleb-associated endoph-thalmitis: clinical features and visual acuity outcomes. Ophthalmology 2002; 109:985–991.
[27] Busbee BG, Recchia FM, Kaiser R, et al.: Bleb-associated endophthalmitis: clinical characteristics and visual outcomes.Ophthalmology 2004;111:1495-1503.
[28] Nagpal M, Wartikar S, Nagpal K:Comparison of clinical outcomes and wound dynamics of sclerotomy ports of 20, 25, and 23 gauge vitrectomy.Retina 2009 ;29:225-231.
[29] Hilton, George F; Josephberg, Robert G; Halperin, Lawrence S; Madreperla, Steven A; Brinton, Daniel A; Lee, Scott S; et al. Office-Based Sutureless Transconjunctival Pars Plana Vitrectomy. Retina:2002 ;22:725-32.
[30] Tan CS, Wong HK, Yang FP, Lee JJ. Outcome of 23-gauge sutureless transconjunctival vitrectomy for endophthalmitis. Eye. 2008;22:150-1.
[31] Doft BH, Kelsey SF, Wisniewski SR, et al.: Additional procedures after the initial vitrectomy or tap-biopsy in the Endophthalmitis Vitrectomy Study. Ophthalmology, 1998;105:707–16.
[32] Shaarawy A, Meredith TA, Kincaid M, et al. Intraocular injection of ceftazidime. Effects of inflammation and surgery. Retina. 1995;15(5):433-8.

[33] Huang SS, Brod RD, Flynn HW Jr. Management of endophthalmitis while preserving the uninvolved crystalline lens. Am J Ophthalmol. 1991 15;112:695-701.

2

Vitrectomy in Open Globe Injuries

Touka Banaee
Eye Research Center,
Mashhad University of Medical Sciences
Iran

1. Introduction

Correct management of traumatized eye is a complicated task needing a sound evaluation of the extent of trauma. An initial history, physical examination and judicious use of Para clinical techniques to determine the extent of injury and construct a prognostic view in mind, are a prerequisite to correct surgical approach to a traumatized globe. The vitreoretinal surgeon is usually not the first physician to see the patient and is consulted for management after a primary ophthalmologist has either repaired an open globe, or has diagnosed the open globe injury or presence of IOFB. For this reason, the primary steps of management of an open globe, although of outmost importance, are not addressed in this chapter.

For a vitreoretinal surgeon to approach an eye with repaired lacerations it is necessary to know the object that has caused the trauma, date of primary repair, procedures that have been done during primary repair, the extent of lacerations, presence or absence of vitreous and tissue incarceration into the wound, and the type of tissues incarcerated. Each of the above data has implications in the management. For example if an eye is traumatized by a piece of wood, then one must consider the probability of presence of wood particles within the eye and the high risk of development of endophthalmitis. In such a case, the surgeon may decide to do an earlier vitrectomy. The date of primary repair is used for timing of the surgery as will be discussed later. And the procedures for example, lensectomy that have been done during the primary repair, may help the surgeon plan about the steps of surgery like the site for placement of the inflow. Knowledge of the extent of laceration and the type and extent of tissue incarceration into the wound will help the surgeon construct a mental model of the condition to predict surgical steps needed and prognosticate the results preoperatively which may help in consultation with the patient and the family.

For a successful vitrectomy to be done, a watertight primary wound closure is necessary. The surgeon must also assess the clarity of cornea and lens (if present) to be sure there will be adequate view of the posterior segment structures for vitrectomy. If there is central corneal laceration, he or she must consult a cornea surgeon to be prepared for placement of a temporary keratoprosthesis and doing penetrating keratoplasty afterwards.

Another piece of data that is very important to have before surgery is the condition of the retina; is it attached or detached and incarcerated. This information will affect the surgical planning much.

Presence of IOFB, age of the patient, presence or absence of signs of intraocular infection, all will affect the timing and planning of a surgery.

2. Mechanism and complications of intraocular fibrovascular proliferation after open globe injuries

It has been shown that scleral lacerations with incarceration of vitreous in the wound have the potential complication of fibrovascular tissue growth into the eye, which will be enhanced by the presence of blood, lens material and inflammation[1]. This fibrovascular tissue can damage the eye by exerting traction on the retina or ciliary body causing tractional retinal detachment (RD) or ciliary body detachment. Growing over the ciliary body the membrane forms of a cyclitic membrane causing hypotony. (Figure 1) To prevent these grave complications, vitrectomy is indicated in every case of trauma that is judged high risk for growth of intraocular fibrovascular tissue[2].

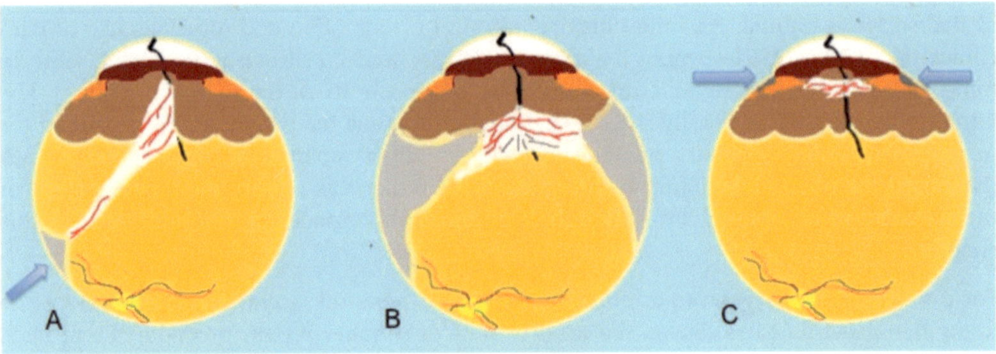

Fig. 1. Fibrovascular ingrowth into the eye can cause many complications: Tractional retinal detachment as a result of fibrovascular tissue growth over the path of a perforating eye injury (A) or in the vitreous base and cortex (B). Traumatic cyclitic membrane results from fibrovascular growth in the anterior cortex of the vitreous body in the region of the pars plicata(C).

3. Indications for vitrectomy in ocular trauma

The following are some of the more common criteria used for performing vitrectomy in an open globe injury:

a. Penetrating eye injuries involving the sclera with:
   i. vitreous incarceration in the wound and moderate to dense vitreous hemorrhage,
   ii. vitreous incarceration in the wound and presence of lens material in the vitreous cavity
   iii. more than minimal retinal incarceration
b. Penetrating eye injuries not involving the sclera with
   i. dense vitreous hemorrhage
   ii. suspected to involve the posterior segment
c. Perforating eye injuries
d. Presence of an (infected or toxic) IOFB

e. Presence of retinal detachment, extensive choroidal detachment or other posterior segment pathologies in need of repair.

Timing of surgery depends on the circumstances. Presence of IOFB or infection mandates early intervention.

a. *Penetrating eye injuries involving the sclera*:
As stated before, scleral lacerations can act as an entrance for migration of fibrovascular tissue into the eye. This can be enhanced if there is a frame for the pathologic tissue to grow on i.e. incarcerated vitreous, and the presence of material with exciting cytokines like blood and/ or lens material. Cleary and Ryan showed that the site of scleral laceration also matters: proliferation is more apt to occur if the wound is in the region of pars plana[3-5]. The primary goal of vitrectomy in penetrating injuries involving the sclera is to halt this process of fibrovascular tissue proliferation by removing incarcerated vitreous, and the blood and lens material present in the vitreous cavity. Secondary goals of surgery are: clearing the media, repair of any associated posterior segment trauma, and prevention of future epiretinal membrane formation or tractional retinal detachment by complete removal of the vitreous.

i. Preoperative considerations:
One of the first considerations in these types of injuries is the indication for vitrectomy. If the media is clear enough for a complete fundoscopy, there is no or mild vitreous hemorrhage, and the site of laceration can be monitored, then the case can usually be safely followed without doing vitrectomy. In other cases without enough view of the posterior segment even if there is no significant vitreous hemorrhage in echography, the surgeon usually errs on the safe side i.e. performing a vitrectomy to be sure there is no additional posterior segment complications to repair.
Visual prognosis is another factor that must be considered when planning for surgery. Although vitrectomy has been performed on eyes with NLP vision[6], the results have not been rewarding. It is judicious to rely on the results of visual evoked potential in eyes with poor vision. If there are some recordable waves in the study, then the eye can be considered a candidate for surgery. Eyes without recordable waves had final visual acuity of hand motion in one study.[7]
Another preoperative consideration is timing of surgery. It has been shown that fibrovascular ingrowth does not grow clinically until the 3rd week after trauma , so surgery must be performed in this time period. There are some surgeons that advocate early vitrectomy i.e. within the first 72 hours after trauma[8]. The rationale behind this type of approach is prevention of fibrovascular tissue formation process from the outset and earlier repair of any associated posterior segment injuries. It is an idealistic type of approach, but may not reach its goal in every case due to the presence of intense corneal edema and congestion of ocular tissues in the first days after trauma, which will hinder surgery by inadequate visualization of the posterior segment and intraoperative bleeding. Also induction of posterior vitreous detachment (PVD), an important step of surgery is more difficult and sometimes impossible early after trauma. Besides, the surgeon may go into the eye without adequate knowledge of the extent of injury due to inadequate preoperative investigations. Many surgeons schedule the operation within the first 2 weeks after

trauma. This lag will allow the cornea to somewhat clear, the ocular congestion to subside and the vitreous to undergo changes that facilitate induction of intraoperative PVD. In this time period there is usually enough time for performing ancillary tests like echography, CT scans, and visual evoked potentials. Some studies have shown that visual prognosis does not differ with the time of surgery and depend more on the type and complications of the trauma itself.[9,10]

Another preoperative consideration to address is adequacy of visualization. With panoramic viewing systems, the probability to have visualization through corneas with central opacities have increased, but a cautious surgeon should always consider the need for use of intraoperative keratoprosthesis and subsequent penetrating keratoplasty in mind and arrange for it beforehand.

Preoperative consultation of the patient and family must include discussion about the prognosis that the surgeon has deduced from preoperative assessments, but also must uncover the degree of uncertainty he or she has about the condition.

ii. Technique of surgery:

Three-port pars plana vitrectomy with the use of wide angle viewing systems is the standard procedure to use for trauma cases.

Transconjunctival sutureless techniques may be adequate in cases that do not need much manipulation near the functional sclerotomies and the surgeon have not planned for scleral buckling. In other cases, the stiffness of 20 gauge probes will be of help, but smaller gauge probes may also do well.

At the beginning of surgery, one of the very important factors to consider is the site of sclerotomies. Doing a sclerotomy adjacent to a repaired wound may cut the sutures of the wound and allow wound gape, or may cause extension of the sclerotomy into the wound. Either situation is difficult to repair. Site of wound is also important from another point of view: for planning the side of sitting of the surgeon. Side of the dominant hand of the surgeon, degree of frontal bossing of the patient and location of the wound all determine the ease of access to the wound and the surgeon must sit in a position to have the best access to the wound itself. There are some cases with the possibility of impact of the traumatizing object to the posterior wall of the globe. In these cases the surgeon must also have adequate access to the posterior impact site, and this is another factor to consider.

To have adequate view of the posterior segment, the surgeon may have to remove the edematous corneal epithelium and wash the anterior chamber. Placement of pars plana infusion cannula is one of the first steps to be taken, but its presence within the vitreous cavity may not be assured due to media opacities. In these cases, one may choose to place an anterior chamber inflow first (in cases with free communication between the anterior chamber and vitreous cavity) and turn the pars plana infusion on when it can be adequately visualized. When the lens is clear, one may use an angled needle for infusion and do a core vitrectomy until the infusion cannula tip can be seen in the vitreous cavity. Having adequate view of the procedure is an important issue that must be met in every case to prevent complications.

In cases with severe hypotony or choroidal detachment, use of a longer infusion cannula should be considered to ensure passing of the cannula through the pars plana epithelium at the beginning of surgery.

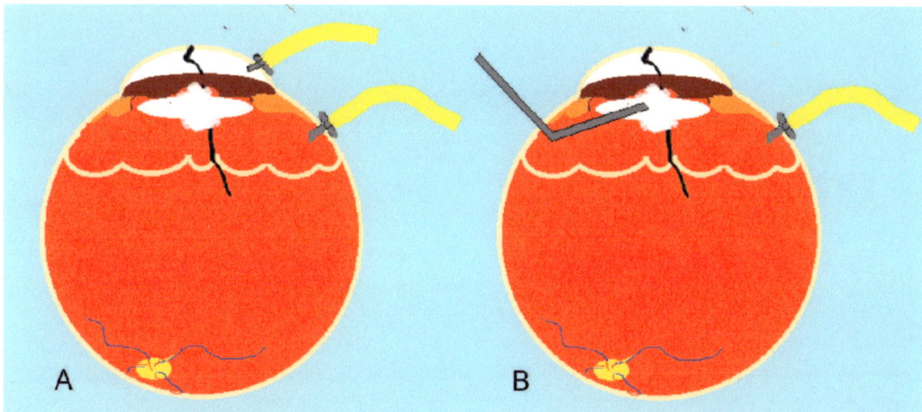

Fig. 2. When the regular posterior inflow tip cannot be visualized at the beginning of the procedure, anterior chamber inflow (A) or a bended blunt needle (B) can be used to make the media clear enough to see the main inflow.

A cataractous lens must be removed through lensectomy. Every effort must be done to save as much capsule as possible. Most surgeons do not place an IOL during the first vitrectomy session in order to place IOL in a more controlled manner: in an eye with stable posterior segment and with accurate calculation of the IOL power[11]. But some have advocated placement of IOL in the first surgery.[12,13]

Another cause for poor visualization during surgery is active bleeding which can be controlled by a. elevating the infusion bottle, b. use of intraocular diathermy, c. fluid/air exchange, d. endophotocoagulation, e. injection of silicone oil, PFCLs, or visco surgical devices, and f. use of thrombin in the infusion fluid[14,15].

In eyes with dense traumatic vitreous hemorrhage, sometimes the RBCs are de-hemoglobinized conferring a whitish hue to the vitreous. There usually are remaining strands of red blood. This view can mimic the retinal surface and sometimes is very hard to differentiate from it. In this situation, the surgeon must work slowly and cautiously; remove the vitreous layer-by-layer and pay attention to the consistency of tissue that is removed. If there is certainty of complete retinal attachment through preoperative assessments, then the situation will be much simpler and the surgeon can work faster.

After removal of the core vitreous, the interior surface of scleral wound should be cleaned of incarcerated vitreous. The incarcerated vitreous must not be pulled out from the wound, but must be trimmed as near to the wound as possible (Figure 3). In limbo scleral lacerations with vitreous incarceration into the wound and a clear lens, one may clean the wound with scleral depression under direct view of the microscope. But this maneuver has the inherent risk of lens capsule touch and cataract formation. Some may do a clear lensectomy from the outset to ensure complete cleaning of the wound. If the lens is clear and hemorrhagic vitreous has been removed, the surgeon can allow less than complete removal of the vitreous from the wound as the risk of fibrovascular ingrowth in this situation will not be high and it seems that the risk-benefit ratio of removing a clear lens vs. complete cleaning of the wound slopes towards retaining the lens. Vitreous base must be

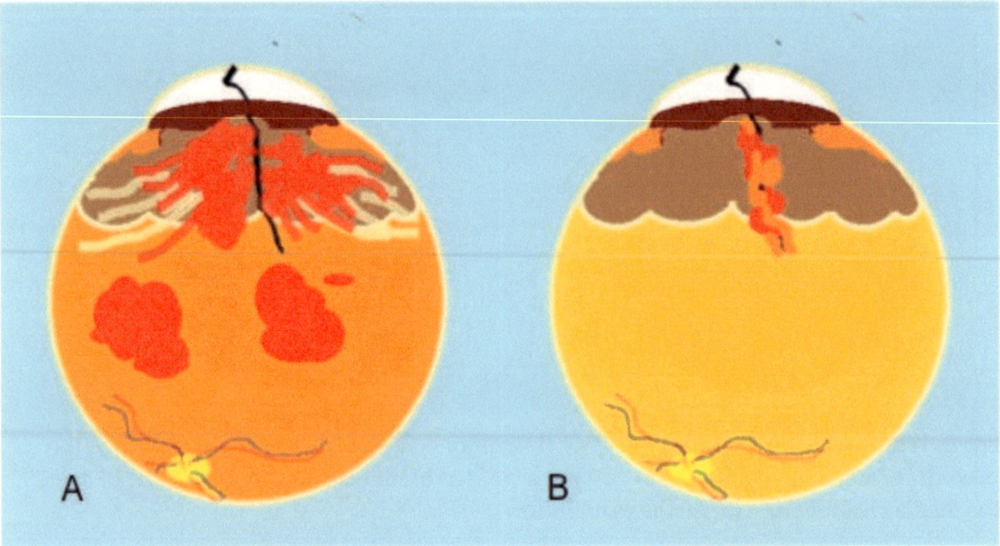

Fig. 3. Corneolimboscleral laceration with incarcerated hemorrhagic vitreous into the wound (A). Trimming of the vitreous incarcerated into the interior of the wound is an important step in this type of surgery removing the scaffold for fibrovascular ingrowth (B).

removed to the extent that is judged to be safe without forming retinal breaks. Induction of PVD is another important step of surgery. Induction of PVD along with trimming of incarcerated vitreous ensures that there remains no scaffold for proliferation of fibrovascular tissue. Induction of PVD is easier when the surgery is done with a time lag after trauma but may be still impossible in very young children.

If there is retinal detachment (RD), both removal of core vitreous, and induction of PVD will be more difficult. Use of PFCLs helps in induction of PVD and stabilization of the retina and in reduction of complications like iatrogenic retinal break formation[16].

The surgeon must identify the type of retinal detachment and its cause. If the RD is tractional, then it is obvious that there is vitreous and retinal incarceration into the wound. If there is rhegmatogenous RD, then the task is to find the causative break.

In cases with retinal incarceration into the wound, if there is minimal incarceration without RD, the case can usually safely be managed with placement of a scleral buckle over the wound without the need to perform retinotomy. But in cases with significant incarceration and RD, retina must be cut near the wound to allow the rest of the retina to reattach. Care should be taken to save as much retina as possible. After adequate relaxation of the retina, perfluorocarbon liquids (PFCLs) can reattach the retina intraoperatively. Retinopexy with endolaser or cryotherapy must be done (Figure 4). Only if silicone oil is going to be used, can retinopexy of a superior retinotomy be deferred.

If there is rhegmatogenous RD, after removal of the vitreous, PFCLs are used and retinopexy applied to the edges of the break.

iii. Use of concomitant scleral buckling

Scleral buckling may be placed for 2 indications:

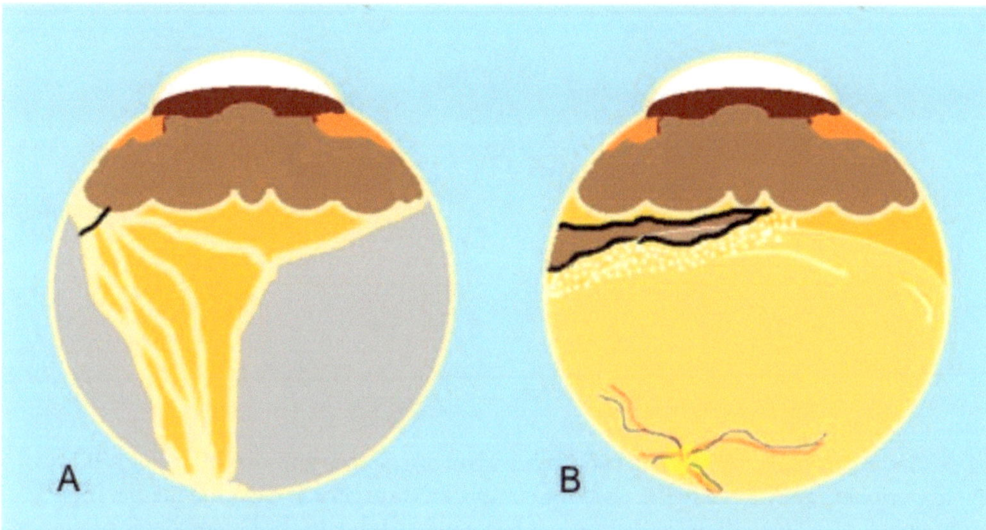

Fig. 4. Retinal incarceration into an anterior wound accompanied by retinal detachment usually needs retinotomy to release the incarcerated retina. Retinotomy must be done as peripherally as possible (A) retinopexy is done after reattachment of the retina under perfluorocarbon liquids (B).

1. Prophylaxis
2. Treatment

Prophylactic buckles are placed when:

a. Media opacities do not allow adequate visualization of the retinal periphery. If the trauma has caused excessive traction on the vitreous base, tractional breaks may have formed in the retinal periphery, and may not have produced RD due to the absence of liquefied vitreous (Figure 5). When the surgeon is not sure of absence of peripheral retinal breaks in a case of severe trauma, she or he may choose to place an encircling narrow buckle to support the peripheral retina instead of doing complicated steps to help visualization of the peripheral retina like penetrating keratoplasty. This complicated surgery, usually does not have good results[17,18].
b. There is no retinal detachment, but there is retinal incarceration into the wound, or there are visible breaks or retinotomies that cannot be adequately supported by endotamponade agents. In this situation one may place a segmental buckle to support the site of pathology, or do encircling buckling.
When buckles are placed in a condition that retinal detachment has occurred, usually support of the offending break or retinotomy is enough, but some prefer encircling buckling.
In traumatized eyes with traumatic cataract, the myopic shift induced by placement of encircling buckle is not a significant issue, as it will be compensated for in the power of IOL that will be placed. Another issue with encircling buckling that has raised some objection to its use is the possibility of induction of choroidal ischemia by encircling buckles[19,20].

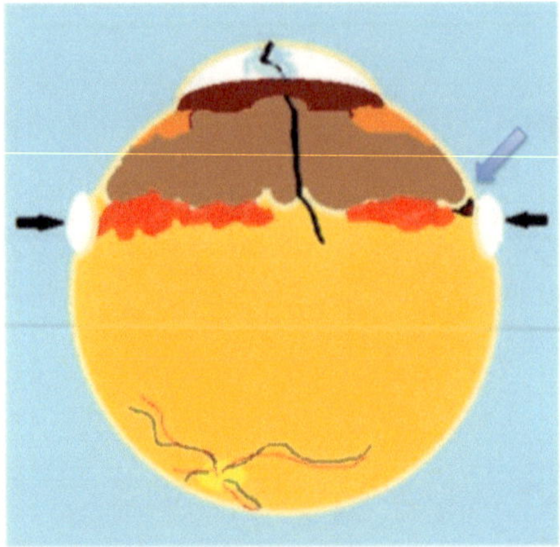

Fig. 5. Placement of a prophylactic band(black arrows) in cases without enough visibility of retinal periphery may obviate the need for complicated surgery to clear the media. Blue arrow points to a small dialysis that cannot be visualized due to the hemorrhagic remnants of the vitreous base and corneal opacity.

iv. Use of endotamponade:
Long acting gases usually suffice for endotamponade in cases with attached retina to support the laceration site while retinopexy takes effect. For cases with detached retina and retinal breaks, or retinotomies, one may choose the agent for endotamponade as a regular case of RD, but I myself prefer silicone oil in these eyes because I believe that reproliferation is more common in these cases and may cause redetachment.[21] I do not want the macula to detach again after primary reattachment.
Inferior retinal breaks and retinotomies must be supported either by an external buckle, or by heavy silicone oil.

v. Management of media opacities:
As stated before, a successful operation needs adequate view of the field. This may not encompass all parts of the retina. If the degree of media clarity is enough to see the inside of the wound, and to induce PVD and be sure that there are no other impact sites and breaks, then performing complicated surgery to restore media clarity is not needed. As stated before, one may choose to place an encircling buckle if he or she is not sure of the absence of peripheral breaks.
When corneal condition does not allow adequate visualization, then one may choose temporary keratoprosthesis placement followed by penetrating keratoplasty, or do the vitrectomy by endoscope (endoscopic vitrectomy). Endoscopes for vitrectomy are not widely available and have a long learning curve so most surgeons prefer the first choice. Anyway, the surgeon and the operating room staff must be prepared for these complicated surgeries beforehand, again accentuating the importance of preoperative evaluation of the eye by the surgeon him/herself.
Another obstacle to visualization of the posterior segment is the condition of the iris which may be adherent to the corneal wound, or be drawn into a limbo scleral laceration. It is preferable to pull the iris out of corneal wound if possible, but this

maneuver may cause wound leak and the need for resuturing. If an adequate pupil is not present, then pupilloplasty must be performed.

vi. Management of accompanying anterior and posterior segment injuries:
In a severely lacerated globe, usually the lens capsule is also damaged and lens material is present in the anterior chamber and vitreous cavity. In these cases, the decision to do lensectomy is straightforward. One important issue is preservation of as much lens capsule as possible for future IOL implantation. If enough capsule for placement of IOL is not present, then the future options for placement of IOL will be: iris supported IOLs, ACIOLs, and scleral fixation IOLs. These eyes usually do not have adequate iris support for placement of an iris supported or ACIOL and scleral fixation of IOL which is a complicated surgery will be the only remaining option.[22,23] Iris diaphragm lenses have been placed in these eyes[24], but recently, glaucoma and corneal decompensation have been reported to occur in long term.
In cases with traumatic cataract with intact lens capsule, preservation of the capsule is simpler.
Lensectomy of a clear lens may be needed in special circumstances like when hemorrhagic vitreous is incarcerated into limboscleral wound and the taut vitreous strands cannot be removed without touching the lens. Another case is for complete cleaning of a limboscleral wound.
Any other posterior segment injuries including retinal breaks, choroidal detachments, and retinal detachments must be addressed during vitrectomy for open globe injuries.
Retinal breaks must be freed of any adherent vitreous and treated with retinopexy and supported by endotamponade. Management of retinal detachment was discussed above.
In case of choroidal detachment, if it is not extensive, then one may leave it untouched. But choroidal detachment that is kissing or so extensive that does not allow the surgery to be performed must be drained. The technique does not differ much from the standard procedure for drainage of postoperative choroidals.

b. *Perforating eye injuries*:

i. Timing of surgery:
All the considerations about timing of surgery in penetrating eye injuries, also apply in perforating eye injuries. Another important issue in perforating eye injuries is sealing of the exit wound, which cannot usually be accomplished during the primary surgery. It takes around a week for a fibrous plaque of adequate strength to form there. So vitrectomy must be scheduled after this time. This lag will also make induction of PVD easier. Sometimes there is a need for earlier surgery, like the presence of endophthalmitis. In this situation, the surgeon must be prepared to have a difficult surgery with intraoperative hypotony, and a protruding globe with extensive conjunctival chemosis.

ii. Technique of surgery:
Perforating eye injuries are open globe injuries that have an entrance and an exit wound. In this type of trauma, vitreous is usually incarcerated in the exit wound and forms a tract between the entrance and exit wounds. Fibrovascular tissue

usually grows on this tract, contracts and causes tractional retinal detachment. Removal of this vitreous scaffold is the basis of doing vitrectomy in perforating eye injuries.

The entrance wound, if scleral, must be treated as in penetrating injuries; cleaned of any incarcerated tissues. Then a deep vitrectomy must follow and PVD must be induced. Induction of PVD is of much more importance than in cases of penetrating eye injuries because remaining vitreous cortex, which is incarcerated at the exit site, will itself act as a scaffold for fibrous proliferation, epiretinal membrane formation and tractional distortion or detachment of the retina. So the surgeon must exert all efforts to induce PVD in these eyes. Induction of PVD may not be easily accomplished by suction over the optic nerve head. Sometimes trimming the vitreous cortex and exerting traction outside the arcades is needed. In other situations, a retinal pick must be used for perforating the vitreous cortex and elevating it. When PVD is induced, the vitreous remains incarcerated at the site of the exit wound. Treatment of the exit wound must include trimming all the vitreous strands incarcerated into it (Figure 6). The vitreous must not be pulled out from within the wound. Usually there is no need for retinopexy around the exit wound, but if there is any doubt about the existence of retinal breaks, then retinopexy is mandatory.

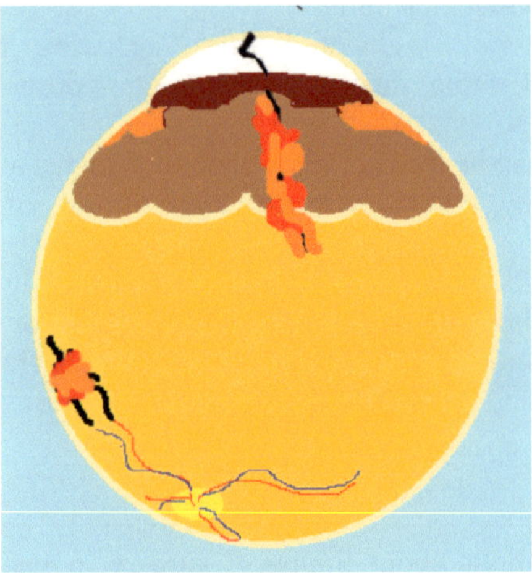

Fig. 6. In perforating eye injuries, trimming the vitreous incarcerated at both the entrance and exit wounds is of outmost importance.

If there is TRD due to retinal incarceration into the exit wound, then one must do circumferential retinotomy around the wound to release the retina and allow reattachment. Use of perfuorocarbon liquids (PFCLs) will attach the relaxed retina and retinopexy can be accomplished by application of endolaser. In such cases my own preference is the use of silicone oil for tamponade; because the risk of proliferation and retinal redetachment is high in these cases.

iii. Use of concomitant scleral buckling:

Scleral buckling for the entrance wound follows the rules for penetrating eye injuries. If the exit wound is at the posterior pole, it is usually supported by internal tamponade agents. Peripheral exit wounds are approached like the entrance wounds in penetrating eye injuries.

iv. Use of endo tamponade:
Choice of the agent used for endotamponade depends not only on the position and condition of entrance and exit wounds, but also on the presence of large retinotomies and use of scleral buckles. For small exit wounds at posterior pole with attached retina, and without entrance wounds involving the retina, long acting gases usually suffice. If retinotomy of entrance or exit wounds is done, one may prefer silicone oil for superior or posterior pole lesions, or heavy silicone oil for inferior lesions.

v. Complications:
One of the common complications during dissection of the vitreous around the wound is retinal break formation. Break formation may also occur at the time of induction of PVD. Inability to induce PVD is considered a major complication in posterior segment traumas as the remaining vitreous cortex acts as a scaffold for proliferation of fibrous tissue resulting in formation of epiretinal membranes or membranes causing instability of the wound or retinotomy. Suprachoroidal hemorrhage which can occur during any type of vitrectomy, may be more common during vitrectomy on traumatized eyes[25]. Avoidance of intraoperative hypotony is very important to prevent this dreaded complication.

c. *Intraocular foreign bodies (IOFBs)*:
Like other traumatic injuries to the eye, occurrence of IOFBs is effectively prevented by adherence to safety measures, because most of them are work related. Some activities like hammering and chiseling have a high probability of producing high-speed projectiles that can enter the eye. War injuries also have a high probability of IOFBs.[26-28] Sometimes foreign bodies are entered into the eye by a larger object impacting the eye such as cilia that enter the eye through penetrating traumas by objects like stone or wood.

i. Preoperative evaluation:
Preoperative evaluation of IOFBs encompasses identifying the following:

a. Material of the IOFB and its magnetic properties
This information is of great help to decide on whether to remove the IOFB or not and to make decision about the technique of removal. It may also mandate a very early surgery due to the toxic nature of the IOFB. This information may be gathered by accurate questioning or even examining the source of the projectile. Ancillary tests like CT scan and echography may also be of some help.
b. Size of the IOFB, which is of critical importance for decision about the technique of removal and determination of prognosis. This can be estimated by fundoscopy or from CT scan images or by echography.
c. Location of the IOFB and its relation to ocular tissues is also much important for planning the technique and the steps of surgery. This information is best got through examination, ultrasonography and CT scans.
d. Risk of infection or presence of any signs of infection; if present mandates surgery as soon as possible even when a non-toxic, non-organic IOFB is

present. Presence of IOFBs has been shown to increase the rate of endophthalmitis.[29]

e. Extent of accompanying ocular damage, which varies widely from minimal to near loss of normal globe architecture. This issue is important in planning the steps of surgery, and prognosticating the case.

ii. Indications for removal:
All IOFBs in the acute phase are candidate for prompt removal because of the potential risk of infection[30]. Beyond that time, an IOFB must be removed if it is toxic or organic, or if it has sharp edges. Iron and copper especially if pure, are the most toxic substances for the eye and must be removed promptly[31,32]. They can cause acute siderosis or chalcosis that can mimic endophthalmitis. Even in the absence of chalcosis, copper has been shown to be toxic to the retinal tissue and induce electrophysiological changes that may be partly reversible upon removal[32]. Plastic, glass and cilia are non-toxic to the ocular tissues and if there is no risk of infection, or they do not have sharp edges, they may be left in the eye.
IOFBs with sharp edges that can injure the retina and have the risk of future RD must also be removed irrespective of their nature.
If there are other ocular injuries in need of a vitrectomy surgery, then removal of IOFB should be part of the procedure.

iii. Timing of surgery:
Some surgeons remove the IOFB during primary repair. This strategy is helpful in preventing the inherent risk of endophthalmitis which is more common when an IOFB is present[33]. Inadequate visualization, inability to induce PVD and risk of hemorrhage are more common with early surgery. Performing surgery on an elective basis, allows the surgery to be done in a more controlled manner with expert personnel being at hand, but the risk of development of infection is more than the previous strategy. Inadequate visualization, inability to induce PVD and hemorrhage may be less of a problem in delayed surgery. Some studies have shown that delayed removal of IOFBs is not associated with poorer visual or anatomical outcomes[27,28]. As it has been shown that prophylactic injection of intravitreal antibiotics reduces the risk of endophthalmitis, if a delayed surgery is planned, intravitreal injection of antibiotics is indicated during primary repair[34]. In one study, this strategy has been followed even in eyes with signs of endophthalmitis i.e. injection of intravitreal antibiotics and doing the vitrectomy in a more controlled condition, and the authors concluded that the results are good enough to consider this strategy as a viable alternative to early vitrectomy[35].

iv. Choosing the technique for removal and appropriate instruments.
This step depends on the material of the IOFB, its magnetic properties, size, location, and presence or absence of traumatic cataract. For magnetic IOFBs, external or internal magnets can be used for removal[36]. External magnets are used only if the IOFB is visible, floating in the vitreous cavity and without a visible capsule. In this case, a sclerotomy about 1.5 times the size of the IOFB is made in pars plana adjacent to the IOFB, and the magnet is placed over pars plana epithelium and turned on while some side-to-side movement is applied to help IOFB pierce the pars plana epithelium.

Most magnetic IOFBs cannot be removed in the above manner, and along with non-magnetic IOFBs must be removed by forceps or baskets.
Baskets are used for small and medium sized IOFBs. Foreign body forceps is used for most non-magnetic and also magnetic IOFBs. But magnetic IOFBs are better elevated from the retinal surface by a rare earth intraocular magnet, and then grasped with the forceps, as the magnet cannot hold the IOFB during passage through obstacles like sclerotomy.
Other techniques for removal of IOFBs like use of snare or catheter have been reported[37,38].

v. Steps in vitrectomy:
If the lens is cataractous and there is the decision to remove it, then lensectomy, via either pars plana or limbal approaches must be done at the beginning of surgery. One must attempt to save enough capsule for placement of IOL; but IOL placement must be deferred until the end of surgery, as one safe place to remove the IOFB is through the anterior segment. Placement of the IOL is usually done at the end of surgery.[39]
A complete pars plana vitrectomy is needed and as much peripheral vitreous as possible must be removed.[26] PVD must be induced, usually with the aid of intravitreal triamcinolone acetonide injection. IOFB removal must be done after induction of PVD because tractions on vitreous strands during removal of IOFB may easily incite break formation, especially retinal dialysis (Figure 7).

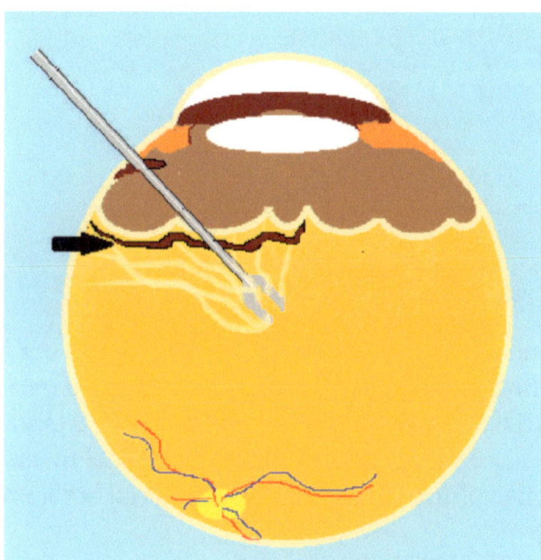

Fig. 7. If vitreous is not adequately removed before IOFB removal, insertion of the forceps or removal of the IOFB through the sclerotomy will cause traction on vitreous base, which may result in the formation of retinal dialysis (black arrow).

If there is accompanying RD, use of PFCLs after induction of PVD will cause retinal reattachment and will facilitate IOFB removal. The surgeon must find the causative break(s) and be sure of their proper management.

vi. Choosing the site for extraction of foreign body: pars plana vs. limbal incision
The surgeon must decide which route for IOFB removal will cause least damage to the ocular tissues. If the lens was cataractous and lensectomy has been done, IOFB

can be removed through a posterior and anterior capsulotomy and through a clear corneal or limbal wound. This way is my preferred method for removal IOFBs if the lens is not present (Figure 8 B).

For removal of large IOFBs through pars plana, the sclerotomy must be enlarged to a large size and a large sclerotomy has a high risk for posterior segment complications like vitreous incarceration and retinal break formation, so one may choose clear lens extraction to remove a large IOFB through a limbal incision.

For small IOFBs, in an eye with clear lens, the pars plana sclerotomy can be enlarged to accommodate the forceps grasping the IOFB (Figure 8 A).

In every case of IOFB removal, the surgeon must examine retinal periphery at the end of operation meticulously.

The site of IOFB impact may be left without retinopexy provided that PVD has been induced and the vitreous has been completely cut from around the impact site[40].

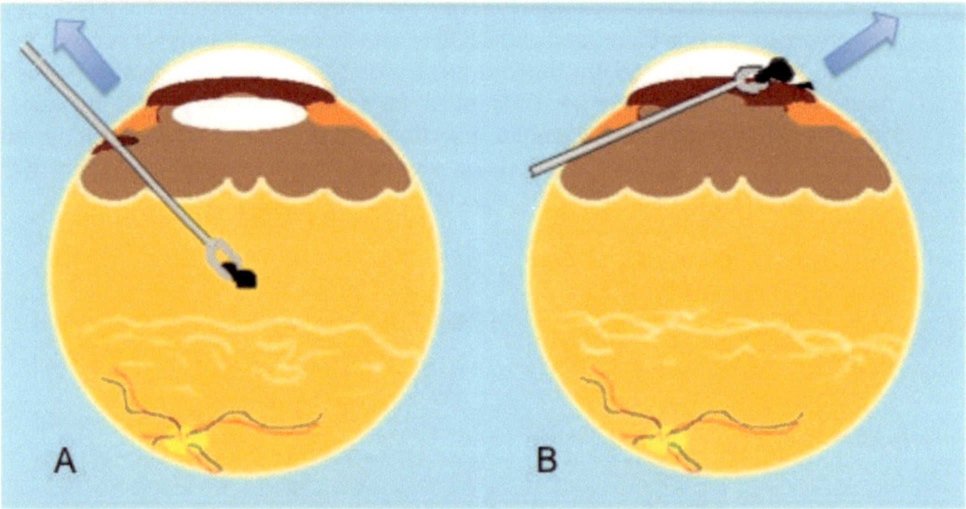

Fig. 8. The sclerotomy is enlarged in phakic eyes before introducing the forceps or basket for removal of the IOFB. Although removal of small IOFBs through enlarged sclerotomy is relatively safe, for larger IOFBs or whenever the eye is aphakic, extraction through a limbal incision seems to be safer. Note that for protection of a normal fovea, the vitreous cavity is filled up to two thirds of its volume by visco-elastic material before removal of the IOFB.

vii. Protecting the normal macula:

In most cases undergoing surgery for IOFBs, the macula is not affected. Maintaining a healthy macula during surgery is the key to good visual prognosis. As there is the risk of drop of the IOFB over the normal macula during various steps of surgery: releasing the IOFB, it's grasping by forceps and extraction through sclerotomy or anterior segment structures, surgeons have proposed various methods to protect the normal macula. Use of PFCLs and visco-surgical devices are some to mention[41,42] (Figure 8).

viii. Complications:

In addition to the typical complications of a vitrectomy procedure, intraoperative hemorrhage and retinal break formation are significant complications that can occur in this type of surgery. If an IOFB is impacted into the choroid, its manipulations have the inherent risk of choroidal hemorrhage. One must be prepared to confront this condition with prompt elevation of IOP and use of PFCLs to prevent sub macular migration of the hemorrhage.

Retinal breaks may form when the IOFB is being released from its attachments to the retina or when attempting to grasp it with a forceps. Traction on vitreous strands is another cause for formation of peripheral retinal breaks. Meticulous surgery and complete removal of the vitreous are key factors to prevent retinal break formation. Postoperative retinal detachment have been reported to occur in eyes undergoing IOFB removal in 6.25% to 32.5% of cases [43-45].

Another reported complication of IOFB removal is late onset RRD[46].

Traumatic cataract is another complication of vitrectomy for removal of IOFBs. If a long or twisted IOFB is to be removed from pars plana, with a clear lens in place, the surgeon must be cautious to avoid contact of the instruments or IOFB with the lens.

ix. Prognosis:

Visual prognosis for eyes with small to medium sized IOFBs is generally good except for cases with direct impact of the IOFB to the fovea, or those developing endophthalmitis. The prognosis for eyes with large IOFBs is more unpredictable because there is not only higher risk of posterior pole impact, but also more surgical complications.[47-49] Presence of preoperative RD also worsens the prognosis.[48,49]

About one third to half of eyes containing IOFBs attain final VA of 6/12 or more[43,45,50].

d. *Endophthalmitis and vitreous abscess*:

Posttraumatic endophthalmitis and vitreous abscess formation is another indication for doing vitrectomy in open globe injuries.

i. Prophylaxis of posttraumatic endophthalmitis:

Cases with open globe injuries are usually hospitalized and receive 3 days of prophylactic systemic antibiotics.[29] Intravitreal injection of Cefazoline and Gentamicin during primary repair have been shown to be only effective for prophylaxis against development of endophthalmitis if the eye harbors an IOFB[34].

In cases that primary repair may be delayed and there is a large wound, intravitreal injection of antibiotics have also been proposed[51].

ii. Timing of surgery:

If there is suspicion of posttraumatic endophthalmitis in an eye with repaired open globe injury, management depends on severity and course of endophthalmitis and the need for vitreous surgery for indications cited above.

In an eye without any other indications for vitrectomy, for example in an eye with corneal laceration, and traumatic cataract without any other posterior segment injuries, endophthalmitis with a subacute course may well be controlled with intravitreal antibiotics. Prompt vitrectomy has been advocated for other scenarios of endophthalmitis in eyes with open globe injuries[52]. Early vitrectomy has the advantage of being able to do the procedures intended for an open globe injury when the media have not become much hazy and halting the fibrovascular ingrowth which is accentuated by the presence of infection.[21]

If there is an acute or hyper acute endophthalmitis in an eye that has sustained open globe injury, then doing the vitrectomy may not be so simple especially when there exists an RD. Doing vitrectomy and complicated vitreoretinal procedures without adequate visualization is very difficult if not impossible. In this difficult situation, the surgeon may opt to quiet the infection by doing a vitrectomy (not a complete vitrectomy but as much as possible and safe) and washing the vitreous cavity with infusion fluid containing diluted antibiotics, filling the eye with silicone oil, and doing a second operation at a later date. Silicone oil is the preferred tamponade agent if there is RD plus endophthalmitis.[53]

iii. Goals of surgery
Vitrectomy for endophthalmitis in cases with repaired open globe injuries is done with 2 main goals:
  a. Control of the infection,
  b. Achieving the goals of vitrectomy in open globe injuries at the same time minimizing the probability of iatrogenic trauma and complications of surgery.

iv. Surgical steps:
Like vitrectomy for postoperative endophthalmitis, it is desirable to get an undiluted sample of the vitreous for laboratory evaluations. But due to the disorganization of ocular structure and probability of presence of RD, one must be very cautious not to make iatrogenic trauma when dry vitrectomy with its attendant hypotony is performed. The infusion is turned on after the sample is taken. It is advisable to use diluted antibiotics in the infusion fluid. As stated above, the surgeon must decide on how complete to do the procedure. In some cases with very poor visualization, the surgeon may decide to do only a core vitrectomy and perform the rest of operation in another session. In this situation, usually the second procedure must not be delayed too much; otherwise fibrovascular ingrowth will take its effect and produce its own complications. In other circumstances, there may be a good condition for performing a complete procedure. Another option in cases with poor visualization is the use of endoscopic surgery[54].
If the surgeon is not sure of the presence or absence of retinal breaks, then use of silicone oil for tamponade, may improve the prognosis.[53,55]

v. Prognosis:
Depends on the virulence of the organism and associated posterior segment injuries. Retained IOFBs and poor initial vision have been found to predict a worse visual outcome[56].

e. *Suprachoroidal hemorrhage*:
Drainage of suprachoroidal hemorrhage in traumatized eyes is similar to other conditions except for the possibility of presence of associated posterior segment injuries needing repair. So one must schedule the operation 5-7 days after the trauma to give enough time to hemorrhage for liquefaction. For access to the globe equator to do drainage sclerotomies, rectus muscles must be caught by bridle sutures. Then a drainage sclerotomy without touching the choroid is placed 9mm from the limbus in the quadrant with the most amount of suprachoroidal hemorrhage. These cases usually have hyphema and cataract in association with suprachoroidal hemorrhage and at the beginning of the operation the anterior segment should be cleaned of

hemorrhage, lens material, and vitreous. For this step usually an anterior chamber inflow can be placed. After cleaning the anterior segment and performing lensectomy of a cataractous lens, a long posterior chamber inflow usually 6 mm long is placed through pars plana. Prior to this step, one may infuse air through the anterior chamber inflow and open lips of the drainage sclerotomy with a forceps to help reduce the suprachoroidal hemorrhage. This maneuver may somewhat lessen the degree of protrusion of the pars plana epithelium and enhance placement of an inflow. The pars plana infusion should be turned on only after its tip has been seen to be in the vitreous cavity. Then with the combined infusion of air and perfluorocarbon liquids, the most complete drainage of the suprachoroidal hemorrhage can be accomplished. The surgeon must always be prepared to face other posterior segment injuries in these complicated cases and must repair them too. One important matter in this situation is that fishing of clot or hemorrhage through the sclerotomy is forbidden and may damage the choroid and the retina. Subtotal drainage of suprachoroidals is preferable to making additional retinal and choroidal injuries.

f. *Dense vitreous hemorrhage without other identifiable posterior segment injuries*:
In a case of open globe injury with dense vitreous hemorrhage and no other identifiable injuries in echography, it is desirable to clear media within a reasonable time usually the first two weeks after trauma to be sure of the absence of injuries that may have been missed in echography like damage to retinal vessels or ciliary body without significant vitreous incarceration.

g. *Removal of Traumatic cyclitic membranes*:
Traumatic cyclitic membranes i.e. fibrovascular membranes covering the ciliary body are one of the late complications of open globe injuries involving the anterior sclera. This complication usually occurs in eyes with scleral lacerations and vitreous incarceration along with vitreous hemorrhage or liberated lens material in the vitreous cavity that have not undergone due pars plana vitrectomy. Another condition that theoretically may predispose to their development is inadequate vitrectomy and cleaning of the wound and vitreous base area. When they develop, they lead to ocular hypotony and can cause phthisis. These eyes essentially do not have worse ocular traumas than others but are lost as a result of delay in surgery. Ocular hypotony after trauma may have other etiologies such as: post traumatic uveitis and cyclodialysis cleft and RD. The first one is temporary and does not persist for more than a few weeks. Cyclodialysis clefts are visible in gonioscopy, which may be very difficult to do in these eyes and ultrasound biomicroscopy is a viable alternative option for their diagnosis.[57] RD can be diagnosed with ultrasonography.
Sometimes the cyclitic membrane grows in the pupillary area to produce a fibrovascular membrane visible through the pupil causing extensive posterior synechia formation.
Removal of these membranes is a demanding procedure. Zarbin et al[58] discussed the technique of dissection for cyclitic membranes secondary to PVR. But traumatic cyclitic membranes are different from anterior PVR. Traumatic membranes usually grow on the anterior hyaloid face over the pars plicata and do not make anteroposterior contraction of the vitreous base. To see the region of pars plicata, the surgeon must use scleral depression and direct viewing through the operating microscope. Another option is the use of endoscopic vitrectomy.

One technique described for their removal includes removal of the center of the membrane and core vitrectomy, placement of radial cuts over the membrane and removal of the remnants with vitrectomy probe. It has been reported that if one quarter of the ciliary body circumference is salvaged, then the IOP returns back to normal. Cases with cyclitic membrane and RD after open globe injury have a poor prognosis.[22]

4. Is there an inoperable eye after trauma?

There are reports of vitrectomy on eyes with NLP. But generally the prognosis is poor[6,59]. Presenting vision has been shown to be the most important prognostic factor in traumatized eyes [60]. So the surgeon must consult the patient about prognosis of an eye with poor vision and both decide about the management.

So if the eye can be closed during primary surgery, vitrectomy can be done. But the surgeon must weigh the risks and benefits of surgery and consult the patient and family about doing the operation.

5. Prognosis of open globe injuries with posterior segment involvement

Generally studies have reported up to 50% final vision of 20/50 or better after vitrectomy for open globe injuries[61].

Several factors have been reported to contend a poor visual prognosis in these injuries including: poor initial VA[60,62,63], initial relative afferent pupillary defect[60], site[63,64] and large size of laceration[60,62,65], presence of intraocular foreign bodies, perforating eye injuries, associated posterior segment injuries[63,64], delay in primary repair[66], and endophthalmitis[62].

6. References

[1] Abrams GW, Topping TM, Machemer R. Vitrectomy for injury: the effect on intraocular proliferation following perforation of the posterior segment of the rabbit eye. Arch Ophthalmol 1979;97:743-8.

[2] Cleary PE, Ryan SJ. Vitrectomy in penetrating eye injury. Results of a controlled trial of vitrectomy in an experimental posterior penetrating eye injury in the rhesus monkey. Arch Ophthalmol 1981;99:287-92.

[3] Cleary PE, Ryan SJ. Posterior perforating eye injury. Experimental animal model. Trans Ophthalmol Soc U K 1978;98:34-7.

[4] Cleary PE, Ryan SJ. Experimental posterior penetrating eye injury in the rabbit. I. Method of production and natural history. Br J Ophthalmol 1979;63:306-11.

[5] Cleary PE, Ryan SJ. Experimental posterior penetrating eye injury in the rabbit. II. Histology of wound, vitreous, and retina. Br J Ophthalmol 1979;63:312-21.

[6] Yan H, Cui J, Zhang J, Chen S, Xu Y. Penetrating keratoplasty combined with vitreoretinal surgery for severe ocular injury with blood-stained cornea and no light perception. Ophthalmologica 2006;220:186-9.

[7] Hutton WL, Fuller DG. Factors influencing final visual results in severely injured eyes. Am J Ophthalmol 1984;97:715-22.

[8] Coleman DJ. Early vitrectomy in the management of the severely traumatized eye. Am J Ophthalmol 1982;93:543-51.

[9] Dalma-Weiszhausz J, Quiroz-Mercado H, Morales-Canton V, Oliver-Fernandez K, De Anda-Turati M. Vitrectomy for ocular trauma: a question of timing? Eur J Ophthalmol 1996;6:460-3.
[10] de Juan E, Jr., Sternberg P, Jr., Michels RG. Timing of vitrectomy after penetrating ocular injuries. Ophthalmology 1984;91:1072-4.
[11] Chuang LH, Lai CC. Secondary intraocular lens implantation of traumatic cataract in open-globe injury. Can J Ophthalmol 2005;40:454-9.
[12] Assi A, Chacra CB, Cherfan G. Combined lensectomy, vitrectomy, and primary intraocular lens implantation in patients with traumatic eye injury. Int Ophthalmol 2008;28:387-94.
[13] Chan TK, Mackintosh G, Yeoh R, Lim AS. Primary posterior chamber IOL implantation in penetrating ocular trauma. Int Ophthalmol 1993;17:137-41.
[14] de Bustros S. Intraoperative control of hemorrhage in penetrating ocular injuries. Retina 1990;10 Suppl 1:S55-8.
[15] de Bustros S, Glaser BM, Johnson MA. Thrombin infusion for the control of intraocular bleeding during vitreous surgery. Arch Ophthalmol 1985;103:837-9.
[16] Desai UR, Peyman GA, Harper CA, 3rd. Perfluorocarbon liquid in traumatic vitreous hemorrhage and retinal detachment. Ophthalmic Surg 1993;24:537-41.
[17] Roters S, Hamzei P, Szurman P, et al. Combined penetrating keratoplasty and vitreoretinal surgery with silicone oil: a 1-year follow-up. Graefes Arch Clin Exp Ophthalmol 2003;241:24-33.
[18] Roters S, Szurman P, Hermes S, Thumann G, Bartz-Schmidt KU, Kirchhof B. Outcome of combined penetrating keratoplasty with vitreoretinal surgery for management of severe ocular injuries. Retina 2003;23:48-56.
[19] Sato EA, Shinoda K, Inoue M, Ohtake Y, Kimura I. Reduced choroidal blood flow can induce visual field defect in open angle glaucoma patients without intraocular pressure elevation following encircling scleral buckling. Retina 2008;28:493-7.
[20] Kimura I, Shinoda K, Eshita T, Inoue M, Mashima Y. Relaxation of encircling buckle improved choroidal blood flow in a patient with visual field defect following encircling procedure. Jpn J Ophthalmol 2006;50:554-6.
[21] Cardillo JA, Stout JT, LaBree L, et al. Post-traumatic proliferative vitreoretinopathy. The epidemiologic profile, onset, risk factors, and visual outcome. Ophthalmology 1997;104:1166-73.
[22] Banaee T, Ahmadieh H, Abrishami M, Moosavi M. Removal of traumatic cyclitic membranes: surgical technique and results. Graefes Arch Clin Exp Ophthalmol 2007;245:443-7.
[23] Ahn JK, Yu HG, Chung H, Wee WR, Lee JH. Transscleral fixation of a foldable intraocular lens in aphakic vitrectomized eyes. J Cataract Refract Surg 2003;29:2390-6.
[24] Moghimi S, Riazi Esfahani M, Maghsoudipour M. Visual function after implantation of aniridia intraocular lens for traumatic aniridia in vitrectomized eye. Eur J Ophthalmol 2007;17:660-5.
[25] Mei H, Xing Y, Yang A, Wang J, Xu Y, Heiligenhaus A. Suprachoroidal hemorrhage during pars plana vitrectomy in traumatized eyes. Retina 2009;29:473-6.
[26] Ahmadieh H, Sajjadi H, Azarmina M, Soheilian M, Baharivand N. Surgical management of intraretinal foreign bodies. Retina 1994;14:397-403.

[27] Blanch RJ, Bindra MS, Jacks AS, Scott RA. Ophthalmic injuries in British Armed Forces in Iraq and Afghanistan. Eye (Lond);25:218-23.

[28] Colyer MH, Weber ED, Weichel ED, et al. Delayed intraocular foreign body removal without endophthalmitis during Operations Iraqi Freedom and Enduring Freedom. Ophthalmology 2007;114:1439-47.

[29] Andreoli CM, Andreoli MT, Kloek CE, Ahuero AE, Vavvas D, Durand ML. Low rate of endophthalmitis in a large series of open globe injuries. Am J Ophthalmol 2009;147:601-8 e2.

[30] Chaudhry IA, Shamsi FA, Al-Harthi E, Al-Theeb A, Elzaridi E, Riley FC. Incidence and visual outcome of endophthalmitis associated with intraocular foreign bodies. Graefes Arch Clin Exp Ophthalmol 2008;246:181-6.

[31] Billi B, Lesnoni G, Scassa C, Giuliano MA, Coppe AM, Rossi T. Copper intraocular foreign body: diagnosis and treatment. Eur J Ophthalmol 1995;5:235-9.

[32] Dayan MR, Cottrell DG, Mitchell KW. Reversible retinal toxicity associated with retained intravitreal copper foreign body in the absence of intraocular inflammation. Acta Ophthalmol Scand 1999;77:597-8.

[33] Bhagat N, Nagori S, Zarbin M. Post-traumatic Infectious Endophthalmitis. Surv Ophthalmol;56:214-51.

[34] Soheilian M, Rafati N, Mohebbi MR, et al. Prophylaxis of acute posttraumatic bacterial endophthalmitis: a multicenter, randomized clinical trial of intraocular antibiotic injection, report 2. Arch Ophthalmol 2007;125:460-5.

[35] Knox FA, Best RM, Kinsella F, et al. Management of endophthalmitis with retained intraocular foreign body. Eye (Lond) 2004;18:179-82.

[36] Chow DR, Garretson BR, Kuczynski B, et al. External versus internal approach to the removal of metallic intraocular foreign bodies. Retina 2000;20:364-9.

[37] Yao Y, Wang ZJ, Yan S, Huang YF. An alternative method of extraction: use of a catheter to remove intraocular foreign bodies during vitrectomy. Retina 2009;29:552-5.

[38] Erakgun T, Akkin C, Mentes J. Management of the posterior segment foreign bodies with a simple snare. Retina 2003;23:858-60.

[39] Azad R, Sharma YR, Mitra S, Pai A. Triple procedure in posterior segment intraocular foreign body. Indian J Ophthalmol 1998;46:91-2.

[40] Ambler JS, Meyers SM. Management of intraretinal metallic foreign bodies without retinopexy in the absence of retinal detachment. Ophthalmology 1991;98:391-4.

[41] Vartanyan AH, Hovhannisyan TA. Application of perfluorocarbon liquid in the removal of metallic intraretinal foreign bodies. Med Sci Monit 2002;8:CR66-71.

[42] Banaee T, Sharepoor M. Foveal protection with viscoelastic material during removal of posterior segment foreign bodies. J Ophthalmic Vis Res 2010;5:68-70.

[43] Soheilian M, Feghi M, Yazdani S, et al. Surgical management of non-metallic and non-magnetic metallic intraocular foreign bodies. Ophthalmic Surg Lasers Imaging 2005;36:189-96.

[44] Demircan N, Soylu M, Yagmur M, Akkaya H, Ozcan AA, Varinli I. Pars plana vitrectomy in ocular injury with intraocular foreign body. J Trauma 2005;59:1216-8.

[45] Wani VB, Al-Ajmi M, Thalib L, et al. Vitrectomy for posterior segment intraocular foreign bodies: visual results and prognostic factors. Retina 2003;23:654-60.

[46] Weissgold DJ, Kaushal P. Late onset of rhegmatogenous retinal detachments after successful posterior segment intraocular foreign body removal. Br J Ophthalmol 2005;89:327-31.
[47] Armstrong MF. A review of intraocular foreign body injuries and complications in N. Ireland from 1978-1986. Int Ophthalmol 1988;12:113-7.
[48] Bai HQ, Yao L, Meng XX, Wang YX, Wang DB. Visual outcome following intraocular foreign bodies: a retrospective review of 5-year clinical experience. Eur J Ophthalmol;21:98-103.
[49] Chiquet C, Zech JC, Denis P, Adeleine P, Trepsat C. Intraocular foreign bodies. Factors influencing final visual outcome. Acta Ophthalmol Scand 1999;77:321-5.
[50] De Souza S, Howcroft MJ. Management of posterior segment intraocular foreign bodies: 14 years' experience. Can J Ophthalmol 1999;34:23-9.
[51] Gupta A, Srinivasan R, Gulnar D, Sankar K, Mahalakshmi T. Risk factors for post-traumatic endophthalmitis in patients with positive intraocular cultures. Eur J Ophthalmol 2007;17:642-7.
[52] Abu el-Asrar AM, al-Amro SA, al-Mosallam AA, al-Obeidan S. Post-traumatic endophthalmitis: causative organisms and visual outcome. Eur J Ophthalmol 1999;9:21-31.
[53] Aras C, Ozdamar A, Karacorlu M, Ozkan S. Silicone oil in the surgical treatment of endophthalmitis associated with retinal detachment. Int Ophthalmol 2001;24:147-50.
[54] De Smet MD, Carlborg EA. Managing severe endophthalmitis with the use of an endoscope. Retina 2005;25:976-80.
[55] Azad R, Ravi K, Talwar D, Rajpal, Kumar N. Pars plana vitrectomy with or without silicone oil endotamponade in post-traumatic endophthalmitis. Graefes Arch Clin Exp Ophthalmol 2003;241:478-83.
[56] Das T, Kunimoto DY, Sharma S, et al. Relationship between clinical presentation and visual outcome in postoperative and posttraumatic endophthalmitis in south central India. Indian J Ophthalmol 2005;53:5-16.
[57] Berinstein DM, Gentile RC, Sidoti PA, et al. Ultrasound biomicroscopy in anterior ocular trauma. Ophthalmic Surg Lasers 1997;28:201-7.
[58] Zarbin MA, Michels RG, Green WR. Dissection of epiciliary tissue to treat chronic hypotony after surgery for retinal detachment with proliferative vitreoretinopathy. Retina 1991;11:208-13.
[59] Salehi-Had H, Andreoli CM, Andreoli MT, Kloek CE, Mukai S. Visual outcomes of vitreoretinal surgery in eyes with severe open-globe injury presenting with no-light-perception vision. Graefes Arch Clin Exp Ophthalmol 2009;247:477-83.
[60] Rofail M, Lee GA, O'Rourke P. Prognostic indicators for open globe injury. Clin Experiment Ophthalmol 2006;34:783-6.
[61] Hill JR, Crawford BD, Lee H, Tawansy KA. Evaluation of open globe injuries of children in the last 12 years. Retina 2006;26:S65-8.
[62] Mansouri M, Faghihi H, Hajizadeh F, et al. Epidemiology of open-globe injuries in Iran: analysis of 2,340 cases in 5 years (report no. 1). Retina 2009;29:1141-9.
[63] Entezari M, Rabei HM, Badalabadi MM, Mohebbi M. Visual outcome and ocular survival in open-globe injuries. Injury 2006;37:633-7.

[64] Kim JH, Yang SJ, Kim DS, Kim JG, Yoon YH. Fourteen-year review of open globe injuries in an urban Korean population. J Trauma 2007;62:746-9.
[65] Lee CH, Lee L, Kao LY, Lin KK, Yang ML. Prognostic indicators of open globe injuries in children. Am J Emerg Med 2009;27:530-5.
[66] Cruvinel Isaac DL, Ghanem VC, Nascimento MA, Torigoe M, Kara-Jose N. Prognostic factors in open globe injuries. Ophthalmologica 2003;217:431-5.

3

Retinotomy/Retinectomy

Touka Banaee
Eye Research Center,
Mashhad University of Medical Sciences
Iran

1. Introduction

First described by Machemer[1] for relaxing the retina in proliferative vitreoretinopathy (PVR) and trauma, retinotomies have nowadays gained new indications. In many cases of proliferative vitreoretinopathy, the retina does not lend itself to reattachment intra operatively in spite of extensive dissection and removal of membranes[2]. In these cases, there seems to be some intra retinal fibrosis causing shortening of the chronically detached retina. In other cases, the retina flattens under perfluorocarbon liquids or air, but suddenly air or Perfluorocarbon liquids (PFCL) tracks under the retina upon movements of the eye during operation. This is due to the presence of a break(s) with edges under traction. In these cases, if there are no visible membranes to be removed, the only option remaining is cutting or removing the shortened retina i.e.: retinotomy or retinectomy. Cutting or removing part of the retina to allow flattening or access to the subretinal space is part of advanced vitreoretinal surgical techniques.

2. Indications & strategies

Relaxing retinotomies:

There are several indications for doing a retinotomy. The first and best known is proliferative vitreoretinopathy (PVR). In this circumstance, retinotomy is done where there is retinal shortening or extensive epi- and subretinal fibrosis that do not lend itself to removal except for at the expense of formation of retinal breaks. This type of retinotomy is called a relaxing retinotomy. As previously noted, a relaxing retinotomy may be needed to stabilize a break edge. Another indication for performing a relaxing retinotomy is to release the retina that is incarcerated into a scleral wound or sclerotomy and cannot be flattened by either external or internal tamponade.

Access retinotomies:

Sometimes a retinotomy is done to have access to the subretinal space either for removal of substances from under the retina or for doing subretinal surgery. The substances to be removed may be:

- Fluids including subretinal fluid, perfluorocarbon liquids, or silicone oil
- Tissues including choroidal neovascularization, subretinal fibrosis or tumors

Indications for performing retinotomy:
1. Relaxing:
- Anterior PVR & intraretinal fibrosis
- Stabilizing a retinal break
- Retinal incarceration into sclerotomy or scleral wound
2. Access:
- Removing materials from subretinal space:
• Fluids: subretinal fluid, perfluorocarbon liquids, silicone oil
• Tissues: choroidal neovascularization, fibrosis, tumors
- Doing subretinal surgery e.g.: retinal pigment epithelial patch graft

Table 1.

3. Principles

a. Relaxing retinotomies are usually done in a pathologic site of the retina. There are a few rules of thumb for performing a relaxing retinotomy:

   i. Always extend the retinotomy into healthy retina usually for a clock hour from either side; do not fear of cutting too much retina, a large, stable retinotomy that provides the possibility of reattachment under long acting gas or silicone oil is always better than a small retinotomy with unstable edge that either leads to redetachment or requires stabilization by another procedure before removal of the silicone oil (Figure 1).

   ii. When the retinotomy is circumferential, the edges must reach ora by an acute angle (Figure 1).

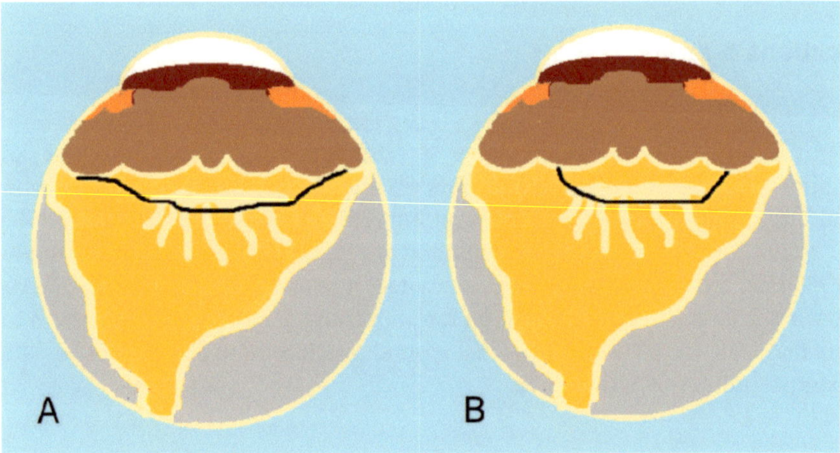

Fig. 1. Correct (A) and incorrect (B) circumferential retinotomies. Note that in the correct technique, the edges of retinotomy extend for a clock hour into normal retina and reach the ora with an acute angle.

   iii. Circumferential retinotomies are always more stable than radial retinotomies (Figure 2).

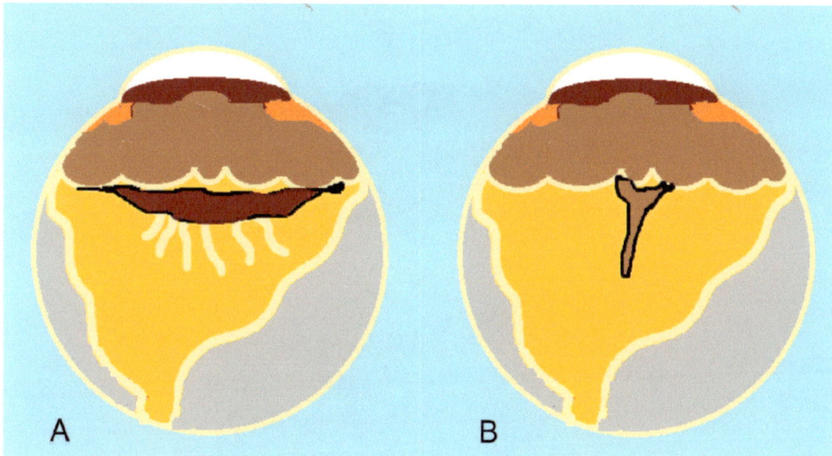

Fig. 2. Circumferential (A) and radial (B) relaxing retinotomies.

iv. In case of retinal incarceration into a scleral wound, the type of retinotomy depends on how much retina is incarcerated and how peripheral is the incarceration. In posterior incarcerations due to perforating eye injuries or intraocular foreign bodies (IOFBs), there usually is the need to cut retina in a circle around the incarceration site. (Figure 4) In peripheral incarcerations, the retina must be cut flush to the sclera to preserve as much functional retina as possible. (Figure3)

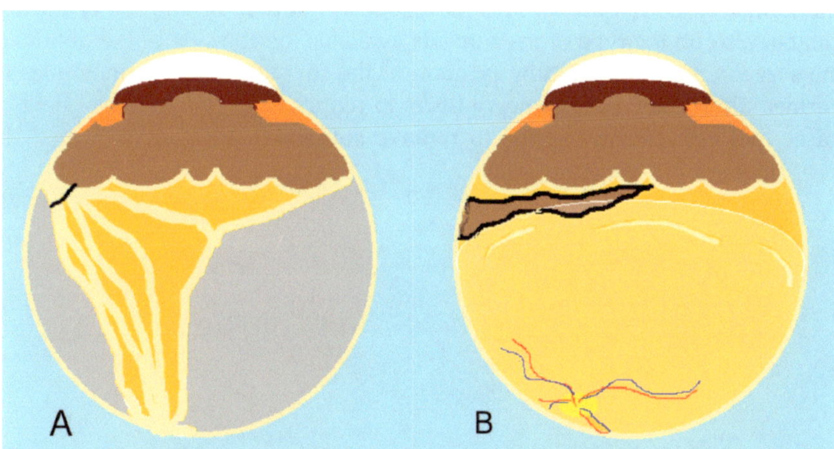

Fig. 3. Retinal incarceration into anterior sclera needs relaxing retinotomy with preservation of as much retina as possible (A). After flattening the retina with perfluorocarbon liquids, the posterior edge of the retinotomy may unexpectedly relax far posteriorly (B).

b. Access retinotomies: Sometimes retinotomy is required to reach the subretinal space, to remove some material or tissues from underneath the retina, or to do subretinal surgery like implantation of tissue in this space[3, 4]. I refer to these types of retinotomies as access retinotomies.

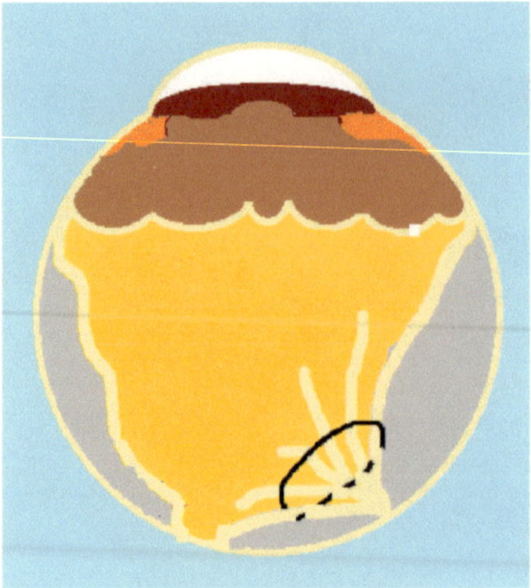

Fig. 4. When retina is incarcerated into a posterior impact site, usually a circular retinotomy around the impact site is needed.

In contrast to relaxing retinotomies, access retinotomies are usually done in a healthy portion of the retina. The size and location of this type of retinotomy, depends on the substance or tissue to be removed from under the retina or the type of subretinal surgery to be done. In these cases, there usually is a preferred site for doing the retinotomy. For example: for removal of subretinal tissues (fibrosis, CNV, and tumors) usually the retinotomy is done in a place to provide access for the surgeon for grasping the abnormal tissue (Figure 5). This may depend not only on the site of the abnormal tissue, but also on the type of instruments available, on the side of the dominant hand of the surgeon and on the sitting position of the surgeon. These retinotomies must be performed along the course of nerve fibers to reduce induction of visual field defects[5]. In cases that retinotomy is done to remove subretinal fluids, it is named drainage

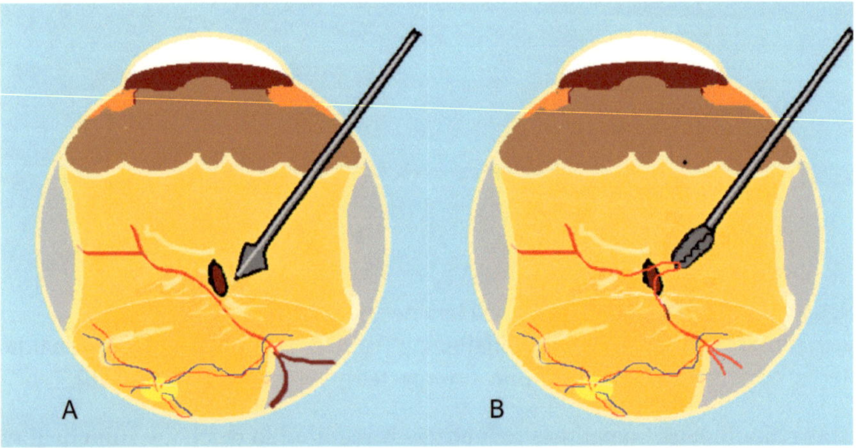

Fig. 5. Retinotomy for removal of subretinal bands (A) is usually done in the superior retina and where it makes access to the subretinal tissue possible. The subretinal band is grasped with a forceps through the retinotomy and gently pulled into the vitreous cavity (B).

retinotomy. This type of retinotomy is usually performed posteriorly to allow complete removal of the subretinal fluid or perfluorocarbon liquids under air[6] or liquids. It is preferably done superiorly to be well tamponaded by routine intraocular tamponade agents, either long acting gases or silicone oil. For removal of subretinal silicone oil, as the oil is usually trapped in the superior and peripheral parts of the subretinal space, the retinotomy is best performed in the superior peripheral parts of the retina over the bubble of silicone oil.

4. Techniques

a. *Relaxing retinotomies*:

1. Anterior PVR:

   Management of anterior PVR is usually done after removal of posterior membranes. The only exception is the central displacement type of anterior PVR that must be removed first to allow access to the more posterior parts of the retina.

   The circumferential contraction type of the anterior PVR is usually amenable to vitreous base trimming along with placement of radial cuts on the vitreous base without much complication. In this type of anterior PVR, dissection is usually successful and retinotomy is not needed.

   The most difficult type of the anterior PVR to manage is the anterior displacement type. In this type of PVR, anterior-posterior contraction of the vitreous base, results in a circumferential fold of the retina at the site of the posterior border of the vitreous base, which is pulled anteriorly, sometimes up to the posterior surface of the iris. Dissection of vitreous base, which must be done circumferentially, is a difficult and delicate job needing a high degree of experience. In these cases some surgeons prefer to defer retinotomy until after extensive dissection of the vitreous base; then if the retina still does not relax enough to rest on the RPE with perfluorocarbon liquids, or by the pressure of air or if multiple retinal breaks have been formed during dissection, retinotomy will be done. Others do retinotomy from the outset with the proposition that dissection of the vitreous base is a time consuming procedure with poor results ending in the formation of multiple retinal breaks that finally necessitates performing a retinotomy. But in my opinion it is not an "all or not" rule. A cautious surgeon guides the operation by looking at the conditions. If the anterior displacement is not complete and the trough of the retinal fold is still visible, vitreous base is amenable to dissection without much complication. In this condition performing a retinotomy is more than needed. But in areas with extensive fibrosis of vitreous base that retinal folds have merged with the fibrous tissue, and the folded retina has formed a closed tunnel, the probability of formation of multiple retinal breaks during dissection is high and performing a retinotomy from the outset may be judicious as it saves time.

   Conventionally, retinotomy is done anterior to 2 rows of endodiathermy to prevent bleeding from major retinal vessels. I myself place endodiathermy spots only over major retinal vessels coursing through the intended site of retinotomy and not as two continuous rows; because tissue injury of endodiathermy can it enhance PVR formation and it is desirable to minimize it.

   A vertical cutting scissors is used for cutting the retina. The vitrectomy probe can also be used to do the retinotomy which may be named "retinectomy". In both

techniques, if the retina is not elevated, there is the risk of damage to the underlying choroid with attendant bleeding. When using vitrectomy probe for retinectomy, this risk can be minimized by a high cutting rate and low aspiration.
In the era that perfluorocarbon liquids and wide angle viewing systems were not available, the surgeon was more confident of reattachment of the retina under air by performing a posterior retinotomy [7, 8]. With the advent of newer surgical instruments and devices, there is a preference to save as much retina as possible and retinotomy is usually performed as peripherally as possible. In cases with anterior PVR, the retina is anteriorly displaced and shortened so after performing the retinotomy, the posterior edge will relax posteriorly and will always rest more posterior than expected by the surgeon. For working so peripherally, usually use of wide angle viewing systems in combination with direct viewing through the microscope along with scleral depression results in a controlled operation. Use of panoramic viewing systems during the procedure encompassing peripheral retinotomy has been shown to reduce the operation time, allow more complete laser treatment posterior to the retinotomy edge and lessen the need for scleral depression[9].
The extent of retinotomy depends on the extent of fibrosis. It must encompass at least one clock hour of uninvolved retina on either side (Figure 1) and must include any nearby iatrogenic retinal breaks. The end of retinotomy at either side must reach the ora with an acute angle (Figure 1). With time, fibrosis of the edge of the cut retina will result in rounding of the ends of the retinotomy. This is an unstable condition resulting in elevation of the edge and possibly redetachment of the retina. When edges of retinotomy reach the ora with an acute angle, this rounding is minimized and usually will not have enough force to elevate the retinotomy edge.
It is preferable to remove the anterior lip of the retinotomy as it is a hypoxic tissue and may cause neovascularization. Some have also proposed that it may redirect the intraocular fluid currents toward the retinotomy, which may enhance redetachment. Fibrosis and exertion of traction on edges of retinotomy is another argument that has been suggested to remove the anterior lip of the retinotomy.
In order to avoid another surgery, YAG laser has been used to perform a relaxing retinotomy in operated silicone filled eyes[10]but has not gained wide acceptance.

2. Retinal incarceration in the scleral wound:
   Ocular injuries can have a variety of presentations and cause various damages to the ocular structures.
   Sometimes retina is incarcerated into the entrance wound (Figure 3). In this circumstance there is usually extensive damage to the retina, as parts of it had been damaged or cut during injury or primary repair of the wound. Usually there is dense vitreous hemorrhage that must first be removed to make the condition visible. If retinal incarceration is minimal and the condition can be managed safely by placement of a scleral buckle, it is preferable to do scleral buckling rather than a retinotomy. But an extensive incarceration can only be managed by retinotomy[11]. Relaxing retinotomy in these cases must be done with sparing as much retina as possible. The surgeon must be cautious when cutting the retina near the wound as hitting the granulation tissue at the wound by instruments, may result in extensive

intraoperative bleeding. Deliberate use of endodiathermy may decrease bleeding from congested retina and surrounding tissues, but one must be cautious in use of cautery to the base of the scleral wound. It may result in the formation of a weak scar and staphyloma in the future.
Another scenario of retinal incarceration into scleral wound is incarceration of vitreous and retina into the sclerotomy of a previous vitrectomy surgery resulting in retinal (re)detachment. In these cases usually a small circumferential retinotomy suffices to relieve the traction. Because of the localized nature of the condition and low lying RD, risk of damage to the underlying choroid and resultant bleeding is high which can be minimized by using the high cut rate and low suction of a high speed vitrectomy system.
Retina may incarcerate at the exit wound, or at the site of the impact of a foreign body. In these cases, if there is no retinal detachment, and the incarceration is minimal the case can be managed by retinopexy around the wound.
But if the retina is detached the best management will be doing a retinotomy around the incarceration site to release the retina (Figure 4), because even if the retina is reattached under the weight of perfluorocarbon liquids, future fibrosis will certainly cause retinal traction and redetachment.

3. Macular translocation surgery:
First described by Machemer[12, 13], in this type of surgery, the retina is detached from RPE by injection of fluid in the subretinal space, peripheral 360 degrees retinotomy is performed and the retina is reattached with some rotation in relation to its natural position. The aim of this type of surgery is to displace the fovea onto a healthier RPE bed. Retinotomy is done for the relocation of the fovea to become possible. It can also be used as an access retinotomy for removal of subretinal CNV and blood.

b. *Access retinotomies*:

1. Drainage retinotomy for removal of subretinal fluid and perfluorocarbon liquids:
There are some cases of retinal detachment and no visible or small peripheral breaks. In these cases, the subretinal fluid does not drain to the vitreous cavity by injection of perfluorocarbon liquids or air. Facing this situation, some surgeons do not touch the subretinal fluid with the assumption that adequate tamponade of peripheral breaks with either scleral buckling or endotamponade will result in the reabsorption of the subretinal fluid by the RPE. If one is not to do scleral buckling, doing adequate retinopexy is mandatory which may be done with cryotherapy without the need for reattachment of peripheral retina. Successful endolaser needs flat peripheral retina and the only option remaining for the surgeon will be performing a drainage retinotomy and draining the subretinal fluid through it.
If the fluid is removed during air/fluid exchange under the pressure of air, fluid will be pushed posteriorly and a posterior retinotomy will be required. A small retinotomy the size to permit soft tip cannula to pass through is usually adequate. Retinotomy is done either by a single cut of the vitrectomy probe or by a sharp needle or MVR blade. Superior location is the preferred site because it ensures adequate tamponade by routine tamponade agents (long acting gasses and silicone oil).

In some cases of peripheral retinal detachment, the macula is attached and a complete air/fluid exchange pushes the subretinal fluid posteriorly which will result in detachment of the fovea. In these cases, doing a retinotomy and drainage of the subretinal fluid will help avoid foveal detachment. An alternative option in this scenario is to remove the perfluorocarbon liquid under BSS and perform a partial air/fluid exchange. If a complete air/fluid exchange is to be done, a small retinotomy is placed near the posterior margin of detachment and the subretinal fluid is drained through it during a slow air/fluid exchange.

This type of retinotomy has several complications including formation of choroidal neovascular membranes and reproliferation at the retinotomy site causing macular traction and redetachment. Damage to the RPE and Bruch's membrane during placement of retinotomy, drainage of subretinal fluid, or retinopexy might have predisposed to these complications[14].

Perfluorocarbon liquids sometimes find way to the subretinal space. This usually occurs during complicated surgeries of anterior PVR with existence of a peripheral retinotomy or large break. The same retinotomy or break can usually be used to access the subretinal space for removal of the PFCL. Besides, subretinal tracking of PFCLs in these cases means that there is residual traction on the edges of the retinotomy or retinal breaks which mandates more dissections or retinotomy. The volume of the subretinal PFCL depends on many factors: the volume of PFCL injected into vitreous cavity and proximity of the causative break or retinotomy to the ora.

Sometimes the cause of tracking of PFCLs into the subretinal space is extensive manipulations and scleral depressions when the vitreous cavity is filled with PFCLs and there is a peripheral break or retinotomy. In this situation, the volume of the subretinal PFCL is small and there is limited access to the subretinal space. If drainage through a break or retinotomy is not possible, the only remaining option will be doing a posterior retinotomy. (Figure 6) It is desirable to do the retinotomy and drainage when the eye is still filled with the PFCL, because in PFCL filled eye, the elevation will usually remain peripheral and localized; but if intravitreal PFCL is removed, subretinal PFCL will settle posteriorly. Considering the location and the small volume of the subretinal PFCL, a retinotomy at posterior pole will be required which will be very dangerous due to the shallowness of elevation.

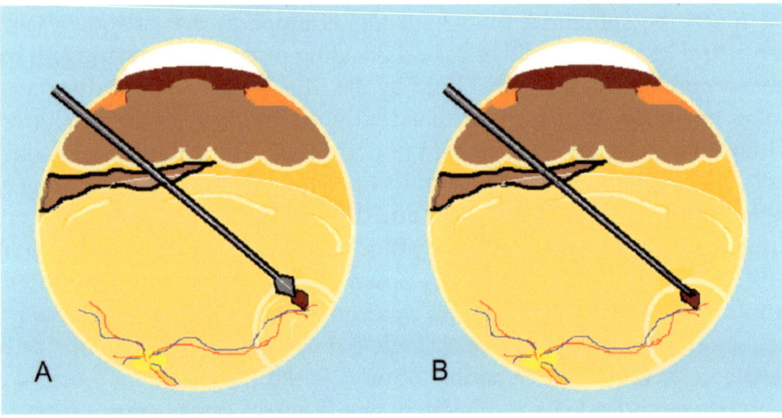

Fig. 6. Drainage retinotomy (A) for removal of subretinal PFCL with a flute needle (B).

Post-operatively with retinal reattachment, and the function of the RPE pump, the retained subretinal PFCL will assume the shape of a subretinal bubble. . Retinal puncture with small gauge needle and active suction of the retained PFCL have been reported[15, 16] Persistence of subretinal PFCLs will result in degeneration of photoreceptors over it[17]. This complication is especially important if the bubble gathers under the fovea. Air/fluid exchange and postoperative upright positioning to push the PFCL to inferior periphery has been proposed for these cases[18].
When the surgeon is not sure about completeness of subretinal PFCL removal, he or she must insist on prone positioning of the patient during the first postoperative day(s) if regular tamponade agents have been used to force the subretinal PFCL migrate peripherally and be trapped as a peripheral bubble.

2. For removal of subretinal silicone oil
Usually these are cases encountered after removal of the silicone oil from within the vitreous cavity, so the vitreous cavity is filled with either aqueous solution or PFCLs and the silicone oil usually accumulates peripherally and superiorly. Removal usually needs a peripheral and superior circumferential retinotomy best done by scleral depression and direct view of the microscope.

3. For removal of subretinal fibrosis and napkin ring
Peripheral subretinal bands need removal only if they hinder retinal reattachment. If they are to be removed, a small radial retinotomy is placed over them and the membrane is grasped with a forceps and pulled through the retinotomy. This maneuver usually results in some small tears around the retinotomy resulting in irregular enlargement of the retinotomy. The best place to do the retinotomy depends on the extent of the membrane, and surgeon's evaluation of the strength and adhesion sites of the membrane. The preferred quadrant of retinotomy also depends on the site of existing breaks, and the tamponade agent that is considered for use. If a heavier than water tamponade agent is considered for use, inferior quadrants will be the preferred site. For regular tamponade agents, superior quadrants are the better choice. But if the site is not matched with the tamponade agent, use of a small segmental buckle to support the retinotomy is prudent.
Usually the membrane gapes away during removal and does not come out in Toto. Total removal of the membrane is not the goal, if tractions are relieved enough to allow the retina to settle under PFCL or air, the procedure is considered enough.
A significant factor to be considered during removal of subretinal membranes is the delicacy of removal. If the membrane sweeps the outer retinal surface during removal through the retinotomy, photoreceptors will be damaged. This will be especially important during removal of membranes near fovea, which may make a good visual result out of reach despite anatomic reattachment. Pulling the membrane along its axis may somewhat prevent this complication.
One of the complications during removal of subretinal bands is subretinal migration of PFCLs. To prevent this, one must keep the level of PFCL well below the edge of the retinotomy. If this complication occurs, the same retinotomy can be used to remove the PFCL. If it is in a peripheral location, a more posterior drainage retinotomy may be needed.
Napkin ring is a fibrous tissue surrounding the optic nerve head preventing normal opposition of the posterior pole. As these eyes usually have extensive PVR and

have peripheral breaks or retinotomies, usually the same sites are used to enter the subretinal space to remove the napkin ring or a 360 degrees retinotomy may be used[19]. Extending the retinotomy circumferentially to have some view of the posterior lesion is usually necessary.

In cases without significant peripheral breaks or retinotomies, a small radial retinotomy can be placed nasally, superiorly or inferiorly near the optic nerve head and used to remove the subretinal fibrosis. But in this technique the surgeon does not have enough view of the membrane and controls the procedure with a view through the retina. In these cases, the risk of damage to the adjacent retina and optic disc components must be weighed against performing a large peripheral retinotomy with its consequences.

4. For removal of subfoveal CNV

Removal of subretinal CNV and blood has been tested in the Subretinal Surgery trials. Others have reported modest visual improvement after removal of massive subretinal blood secondary to CNV[20]. This technique is useful mostly in type 2 CNVs i.e.: membranes over the RPE and under the retina. In type 1 CNVs, the membrane is below the RPE and the RPE must be sacrificed for its removal which will result in atrophy of the overlying fovea[21,22]. To prevent this complication, multiple attempts have been done to transplant RPE with or without underlying choroid[23].

Retina is attached in these cases and for doing the procedure, the first step is induction of RD by injection of BSS into the subretinal space, a procedure called hydro-dissection of the retina. This step is usually done with small gauge needles or cannulas[24,25]. (Figure 7)

The subretinal space can be reached through either a large peripheral retinotomy[26] (Figure 7) or a smaller posterior retinotomy[23]. In cases with large peripheral retinotomies, one may choose to rotate the retina in order to relocate the fovea onto a healthier RPE (macular translocation surgery)[26].

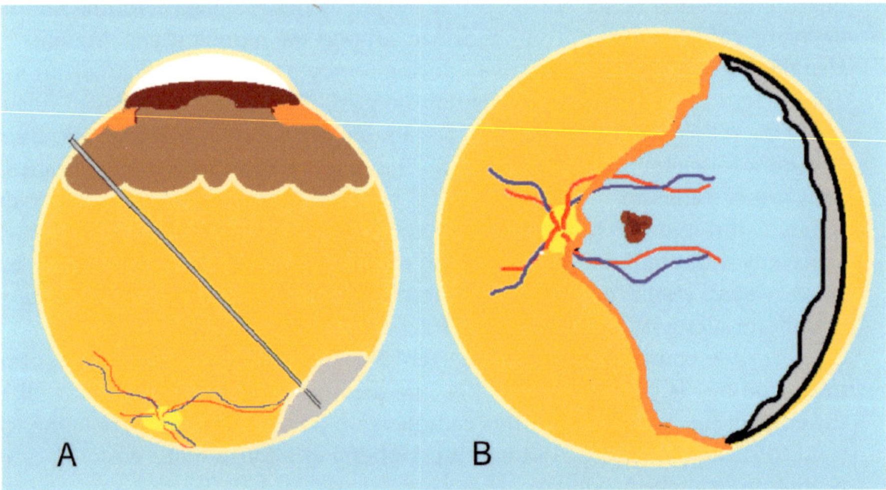

Fig. 7. Retina is detached by infusion of fluid into the subretinal space (A) and a large peripheral access retinotomy is done to reach the CNV (B).

5. For biopsy or removal of subretinal tumors
   Retinotomies have been done to aspirate and biopsy choroidal tumors[27-30]. Intraocular tumor biopsy via a small retinotomy has been reported.[31]

6. For removal of other materials:
   Sub macular hard exudates in diabetic eyes have been removed through a parafoveal small retinotomy[32].Cysticercosis and other larvae[33-35], and blood clot[36] (dissolved by tPA) have all been removed from subretinal space through a retinotomy.
   Removal of subretinal blood loculated in the posterior pole is usually done through a parafoveal retinotomy[36], but removal of extensive subretinal blood, usually needs intravitreal tPA injection followed by vitrectomy surgery 12-24 hours later and peripheral retinotomy with intra-operative drainage of subretinal fluid using PFCLs. Tamponade with long acting gases is employed for further postoperative drainage of the subretinal blood[37].

7. For doing subretinal surgery:
   Different techniques of RPE transplantation or neuroretinal transplantation have been performed after removal of a CNV[21,22,38,39]. Subretinal visual prostheses must be implanted through a retinotomy[40].

5. Extent & determination of adequacy

In case of access retinotomies, the least amount of retinotomy that permits adequate access, view and successful performance without induction of undue complications is done. In cases of relaxing retinotomy, determination of adequacy depends on:

a. adequate release of pathologic tractions to permit retinal reattachment under air or PFCLs
b. stable edge design
c. absence of nearby breaks

6. Management of retinotomy: Adjunctive scleral buckling, retinopexy, internal tamponade

Peripheral retinotomies usually need tamponade, either internal or external. When the site of retinotomy is judged to be inadequately supported by the internal tamponade agent, one may choose to use both.

Some studies have found similar results for silicone oil or gas tamponade[41] in eyes undergoing retinotomy, but other studies advocate use of silicone oil[42]. Presence of relaxing retinotomy seems not to affect the initial outcome in gas filled eyes, but it reduces the need for reoperation if silicone oil is used for tamponade[42]. Inferior retinotomies may best be managed by heavy silicone oils, of which many newer agents are under development[43].

Retinopexy is needed for large peripheral relaxing retinotomies. It can be performed during operation or post-operatively if the retinotomy is adequately supported by silicone oil. Usually 3-4 rows of barrier laser spots are placed posterior to the retinotomy. Delayed completion of the barrage to 360 degrees prior to silicone oil removal, has been shown to reduce redetachment rate after silicone oil removal in eyes that had underwent vitrectomy surgery for PVR[44].

Small posterior retinotomies may be left without retinopexy[5,16].

7. Staged operation

Staged operation have been proposed to improve the results of surgery in cases with severe PVR[45]. In this strategy, one may do the least surgery that can reattach most of the retina under silicone oil. Then during the second procedure, retinotomy will be completed and a third procedure is planned for silicone oil removal.

8. Complications

a. Intraoperative

   Intraoperative hemorrhage is one of the major complications[46] that can be prevented by placement of endodiathermy spots and avoiding damage to the choroid.

   Migration of perfluorocarbon liquids into the subretinal space is a complication of large retinotomies (more than 120 degrees) especially frequent in 360 degrees retinotomies. In one series the authors did not find any difference between two different types of PFCL in terms of subretinal migration[47].

   Another complication of large retinotomies is retinal slippage during air fluid exchange. This complication results from the fluid meniscus between PFCL and gas bubble tracking under the retina causing a shallow peripheral detachment, which under the pressure of air and continuous removal of the intravitreal fluid and PFCL will migrate posteriorly with attachment of the most peripheral parts under air. This reattached peripheral part does not sit on its real position due to the presence of a detached part of the retina posteriorly and sits on a more posterior location, a process called retinal slippage. To avoid this complication, slow air fluid exchange with complete removal of fluid layer over PFCL before removal of PFCL itself is advocated[48]. Another resolution is direct exchange of PFCL with silicone oil. In this technique the fluid over PFCL must be totally removed first too, but because of a more clear view of the process, this goal may be easier to achieve.

b. Postoperative:

   Redetachment due to reproliferation is a major cause for failure of surgery. It depends on the extent of retinotomy and has been reported to occur in 18% to 100 % of cases.[1,42,46,49-51]

   Reproliferation has been reported in up to 50% of eyes with 360 degree retinotomy leading to redetachment in 30% of cases[46].

   Hypotony is another frequent complication of retinotomy that has been reported in up to 43% of cases and is a cause for failure of surgery[8, 51-54]. In eyes judged to be at high risk of hypotony, removal of lens and IOL and making the eye aphakic along with the use of silicone oil have been advocated[55].

   Choroidal neovascularization has been reported to occur as a complication of access retinotomies[56,57].

   Another unexpected complication of large retinotomies is earlier emulsification of silicone oil[58].

The need for performing relaxing retinotomy had been associated with worse visual results in one series[59]. Although some reports have reported correlation between the extent of retinotomy and visual results[49], some others have found no such association[42, 52,53,60].

Visual prognosis is usually limited for cases undergoing relaxing retinotomies for PVR[49,52,53,59,61,62]. Superior retinotomies have been found to have better prognosis[52], possibly due to more complete tamponade with conventional tamponade agents. Also circumferential retinotomies have been reported to be associated with a better visual outcome than radial retinotomies[53].

9. References

[1] Machemer R. Retinotomy. Am J Ophthalmol 1981;92(6):768-74.

[2] Tsui I, Schubert HD. Retinotomy and silicone oil for detachments complicated by anterior inferior proliferative vitreoretinopathy. Br J Ophthalmol 2009;93(9):1228-33.

[3] Kaplan HJ, Tezel TH, Berger AS, Wolf ML, Del Priore LV. Human photoreceptor transplantation in retinitis pigmentosa. A safety study. Arch Ophthalmol 1997;115(9):1168-72.

[4] Augustin AJ, Grus FH, Koch F, Spitznas M. Detection of eicosanoids in epiretinal membranes of patients suffering from proliferative vitreoretinal diseases. Br J Ophthalmol 1997;81(1):58-60.

[5] Verma LK, Peyman GA, Wafapoor H, Greve MD, Millsap CM, Adile SL. An analysis of posterior segment complications after vitrectomy using the perfluorocarbon perfluoroperhydrophenanthrene (Vitreon). Vitreon Collaborative Study. Ophthalmic Surg 1995;26(1):29-33.

[6] Larrison WI, Frederick AR, Jr., Peterson TJ, Topping TM. Posterior retinal folds following vitreoretinal surgery. Arch Ophthalmol 1993;111(5):621-5.

[7] Gremillion CM, Jr., Peyman GA. Posterior relaxing retinotomy. Ophthalmic Surg 1989;20(9):655-7.

[8] Alturki WA, Peyman GA, Paris CL, Blinder KJ, Desai UR, Nelson NC, Jr. Posterior relaxing retinotomies: analysis of anatomic and visual results. Ophthalmic Surg 1992;23(10):685-8.

[9] Lesnoni G, Billi B, Rossi T, Stirpe M. The use of panoramic viewing system in relaxing retinotomy and retinectomy. Retina 1997;17(3):186-90.

[10] Haut J, Le Mer Y, Monin C, Moulin F, Colliac JP. Twenty-five cases of relaxing retinotomy using a nanosecond Nd Yag laser (Yag-retinotomy). Graefes Arch Clin Exp Ophthalmol 1989;227(4):312-4.

[11] Zhang MN, Jiang CH. 360-degree retinectomy for severe ocular rupture. Chin J Traumatol 2005;8(6):323-7.

[12] Machemer R, Steinhorst UH. Retinal separation, retinotomy, and macular relocation: I. Experimental studies in the rabbit eye. Graefes Arch Clin Exp Ophthalmol 1993;231(11):629-34.

[13] Machemer R, Steinhorst UH. Retinal separation, retinotomy, and macular relocation: II. A surgical approach for age-related macular degeneration? Graefes Arch Clin Exp Ophthalmol 1993;231(11):635-41.

[14] Lewis H, Aaberg TM, Abrams GW, McDonald HR, Williams GA, Mieler WF. Subretinal membranes in proliferative vitreoretinopathy. Ophthalmology 1989;96(9):1403-14; discussion 14-5.
[15] Roth DB, Sears JE, Lewis H. Removal of retained subfoveal perfluoro-n-octane liquid. Am J Ophthalmol 2004;138(2):287-9.
[16] Garcia-Arumi J, Castillo P, Lopez M, Boixadera A, Martinez-Castillo V, Pimentel L. Removal of retained subretinal perfluorocarbon liquid. Br J Ophthalmol 2008;92(12):1693-4.
[17] Tewari A, Eliott D, Singh CN, Garcia-Valenzuela E, Ito Y, Abrams GW. Changes in retinal sensitivity from retained subretinal perfluorocarbon liquid. Retina 2009;29(2):248-50.
[18] Le Tien V, Pierre-Kahn V, Azan F, Renard G, Chauvaud D. Displacement of retained subfoveal perfluorocarbon liquid after vitreoretinal surgery. Arch Ophthalmol 2008;126(1):98-101.
[19] Tabandeh H, Callejo SA, Rosa RH, Jr., Flynn HW, Jr. Subretinal "napkin-ring" membrane in proliferative vitreoretinopathy. Arch Ophthalmol 2000;118(9):1287-9.
[20] Fine HF, Iranmanesh R, Del Priore LV, et al. Surgical outcomes after massive subretinal hemorrhage secondary to age-related macular degeneration. Retina;30(10):1588-94.
[21] Cereda MG, Parolini B, Bellesini E, Pertile G. Surgery for CNV and autologous choroidal RPE patch transplantation: exposing the submacular space. Graefes Arch Clin Exp Ophthalmol;248(1):37-47.
[22] Degenring RF, Cordes A, Schrage NF. Autologous translocation of the retinal pigment epithelium and choroid in the treatment of neovascular age-related macular degeneration. Acta Ophthalmol.
[23] Williams DF, Grand MG, Thomas MA. Trans-pars plana vitrectomy in conjunction with scleral buckling procedures for complicated retinal detachment. Int Ophthalmol Clin 1992;32(2):165-71.
[24] Loewenstein JI, Hogan RN, Jakobiec FA. Osseous metaplasia in a preretinal membrane. Arch Ophthalmol 1997;115(1):117-9.
[25] Kubota A, Harino S, Ohji M, Tano Y. Modified technique to create retinal detachment during macular translocation surgery. Am J Ophthalmol 2003;135(1):105-6.
[26] Ninomiya Y, Lewis JM, Hasegawa T, Tano Y. Retinotomy and foveal translocation for surgical management of subfoveal choroidal neovascular membranes. Am J Ophthalmol 1996;122(5):613-21.
[27] Fastenberg DM, Finger PT, Chess Q, Koizumi JH, Packer S. Vitrectomy retinotomy aspiration biopsy of choroidal tumors. Am J Ophthalmol 1990;110(4):361-5.
[28] Peyman GA. Vitrectomy retinotomy aspiration biopsy of choroidal tumors. Am J Ophthalmol 1991;111(1):121.
[29] Garcia-Arumi J, Sararols L, Martinez V, Corcostegui B. Vitreoretinal surgery and endoresection in high posterior choroidal melanomas. Retina 2001;21(5):445-52.
[30] Ahmadabadi MN, Karkhaneh R, Roohipoor R, Tabatabai A, Alimardani A. Clinical presentation and outcome of chorioretinitis sclopetaria: a case series study. Injury;41(1):82-5.
[31] Akgul H, Otterbach F, Bornfeld N, Jurklies B. Intraocular biopsy using special forceps: a new instrument and refined surgical technique. Br J Ophthalmol;95(1):79-82.

[32] Takaya K, Suzuki Y, Mizutani H, Sakuraba T, Nakazawa M. Long-term results of vitrectomy for removal of submacular hard exudates in patients with diabetic maculopathy. Retina 2004;24(1):23-9.
[33] Lerdvitayasakul R, Lawtiantong T. Removal of submacular cysticercosis: a case report. J Med Assoc Thai 1991;74(12):675-8.
[34] Aras C, Arici C, Akar S, et al. Peeling of internal limiting membrane during vitrectomy for complicated retinal detachment prevents epimacular membrane formation. Graefes Arch Clin Exp Ophthalmol 2009;247(5):619-23.
[35] de Souza OF, Sakamoto T, Kimura H, et al. Inhibition of experimental proliferative vitreoretinopathy in rabbits by suramin. Ophthalmologica 1995;209(4):212-6.
[36] Peyman GA, Nelson NC, Jr., Alturki W, et al. Tissue plasminogen activating factor assisted removal of subretinal hemorrhage. Ophthalmic Surg 1991;22(10):575-82.
[37] Oshima Y, Ohji M, Tano Y. Pars plana vitrectomy with peripheral retinotomy after injection of preoperative intravitreal tissue plasminogen activator: a modified procedure to drain massive subretinal haemorrhage. Br J Ophthalmol 2007;91(2):193-8.
[38] Das T, del Cerro M, Jalali S, et al. The transplantation of human fetal neuroretinal cells in advanced retinitis pigmentosa patients: results of a long-term safety study. Exp Neurol 1999;157(1):58-68.
[39] MacLaren RE, Uppal GS, Balaggan KS, et al. Autologous transplantation of the retinal pigment epithelium and choroid in the treatment of neovascular age-related macular degeneration. Ophthalmology 2007;114(3):561-70.
[40] Hegazy HM, Peyman GA, Liang C, Unal MH, Molinari LC, Kazi AA. Use of perfluorocarbon liquids, silicone oil, and 5-fluorouracil in the management of experimental PVR. Int Ophthalmol 1998;22(4):239-46.
[41] Blumenkranz MS, Azen SP, Aaberg T, et al. Relaxing retinotomy with silicone oil or long-acting gas in eyes with severe proliferative vitreoretinopathy. Silicone Study Report 5. The Silicone Study Group. Am J Ophthalmol 1993;116(5):557-64.
[42] Tseng JJ, Barile GR, Schiff WM, Akar Y, Vidne-Hay O, Chang S. Influence of relaxing retinotomy on surgical outcomes in proliferative vitreoretinopathy. Am J Ophthalmol 2005;140(4):628-36.
[43] Rizzo S, Romagnoli MC, Genovesi-Ebert F, Belting C. Surgical results of heavy silicone oil HWS-45 3000 as internal tamponade for inferior retinal detachment with PVR: a pilot study. Graefes Arch Clin Exp Ophthalmol;249(3):361-7.
[44] Laidlaw DA, Karia N, Bunce C, Aylward GW, Gregor ZJ. Is prophylactic 360-degree laser retinopexy protective? Risk factors for retinal redetachment after removal of silicone oil. Ophthalmology 2002;109(1):153-8.
[45] Williamson TH, Gupta B. Planned delayed relaxing retinotomy for proliferative vitreoretinopathy. Ophthalmic Surg Lasers Imaging;41(1):31-4.
[46] Federman JL, Eagle RC, Jr. Extensive peripheral retinectomy combined with posterior 360 degrees retinotomy for retinal reattachment in advanced proliferative vitreoretinopathy cases. Ophthalmology 1990;97(10):1305-20.
[47] Garcia-Valenzuela E, Ito Y, Abrams GW. Risk factors for retention of subretinal perfluorocarbon liquid in vitreoretinal surgery. Retina 2004;24(5):746-52.
[48] Li KK, Wong D. Avoiding retinal slippage during macular translocation surgery with 360 retinotomy. Graefes Arch Clin Exp Ophthalmol 2008;246(5):649-51.

[49] Iverson DA, Ward TG, Blumenkranz MS. Indications and results of relaxing retinotomy. Ophthalmology 1990;97(10):1298-304.

[50] Han DP, Rychwalski PJ, Mieler WF, Abrams GW. Management of complex retinal detachment with combined relaxing retinotomy and intravitreal perfluoro-n-octane injection. Am J Ophthalmol 1994;118(1):24-32.

[51] Banaee T, Hosseini SM, Eslampoor A, Abrishami M, Moosavi M. Peripheral 360 degrees retinectomy in complex retinal detachment. Retina 2009;29(6):811-8.

[52] Han DP, Lewis MT, Kuhn EM, et al. Relaxing retinotomies and retinectomies. Surgical results and predictors of visual outcome. Arch Ophthalmol 1990;108(5):694-7.

[53] Morse LS, McCuen BW, 2nd, Machemer R. Relaxing retinotomies. Analysis of anatomic and visual results. Ophthalmology 1990;97(5):642-7; discussion 7-8.

[54] Ichibe M, Yoshizawa T, Funaki S, et al. Severe hypotony after macular translocation surgery with 360-degree retinotomy. Am J Ophthalmol 2002;134(1):139-41.

[55] Tseng JJ, Schiff WM, Barile GR, et al. Influence of postoperative lens status on intraocular pressure in proliferative vitreoretinopathy. Am J Ophthalmol 2009;147(5):875-85, 85 e1-2.

[56] Richards SC, Maberley AL. Complications of retinotomies for subretinal fluid drainage. Can J Ophthalmol 1993;28(1):24-7.

[57] McCannel CA, Syrquin MG, Schwartz SD. Submacular surgery complicated by a choroidal neovascular membrane at the retinotomy site. Am J Ophthalmol 1996;122(5):737-9.

[58] Gungel H, Menceoglu Y, Yildiz B, Akbulut O. Fourier transform infrared and 1h nuclear magnetic resonance spectroscopic findings of silicone oil removed from eyes and the relationship of emulsification with retinotomy and glaucoma. Retina 2005;25(3):332-8.

[59] McDonald HR, Johnson RN, Madeira D, Schatz H. Surgical results for proliferative vitreoretinopathy. Eur J Ophthalmol 1994;4(4):211-17.

[60] Bovey EH, De Ancos E, Gonvers M. Retinotomies of 180 degrees or more. Retina 1995;15(5):394-8.

[61] Scott IU, Murray TG, Flynn HW, Jr., Feuer WJ, Schiffman JC. Outcomes and complications associated with giant retinal tear management using perfluoro-n-octane. Ophthalmology 2002;109(10):1828-33.

[62] Scott IU, Flynn HW, Jr., Murray TG, Feuer WJ. Outcomes of surgery for retinal detachment associated with proliferative vitreoretinopathy using perfluoro-n-octane: a multicenter study. Am J Ophthalmol 2003;136(3):454-63.

4

Small Gauge Pars Plana Vitrectomy

Rupan Trikha, Nicole Beharry and David G. Telander
Retina Consultants, Little Silver, NJ
University of California, Davis Medical Center
USA

1. Introduction

Although the history of ophthalmic surgery can be dated back thousands of years with operations to treat cataracts, surgery involving the vitreous cavity has only been reported for less than 50 years. The initial description of major vitreous surgery was introduced by David Kasner in 1969 (Kasner, 1969). He described excision removal of the vitreous using a sponge and scissors, under an open sky technique for removal of dense vitreous opacities secondary to amyloidosis. The major problems with this technique including the need for a corneal transplant, lack of control of intraocular pressure (IOP) during surgery, and significant vitreous traction during removal, were addressed by the development of closed intraocular vitreous surgery.

2. Historical perspective

Pars Plana Vitrectomy (PPV) was first developed in 1970 by Robert Machemer. This novel technique provided a closed system for surgical removal of vitreous with control of IOP. The initial device was a 17-gauge (1.42 mm) instrument that combined a vitreous cutter, infusion, and aspiration, and utilized 2.3 mm scleral incision (Fabian & Moisseiev, 2011). O'Malley and Heintz separated the components of vitreous cutting, infusion, and illumination and developed the first 20-gauge, 3-port vitrectomy system (O'Malley & Heintz, 1975). Improvements in technique and instrument design quickly led to the development of the three port vitrectomy system, with lightweight, reusable, pneumatic and electric cutters. For over thirty years, PPV was performed using a 20-gauge, three port system for nearly all vitreoretinal surgery.

As 20-gauge PPV became more widely used, a number of complications became apparent. A major problem was the development of iatrogenic retinal breaks, specifically those at the sclerotomy site. This was felt to be related to repeated passage of instruments though the sclerotomy and vitreous base, with resultant retinal traction and tear formation. Machemer and Hickingbotham introduced a 20-gauge cannula system that was inserted into the sclerotomy for the duration of the surgery, allowing for easier passage of instruments and reducing traction at the vitreous base (Machemer & Hickingbotham, 1985). As experience with 20-gauge PPV increased, a variety of self-sealing 20-gauge incisions were developed to help reduce surgical time, and to improve intraoperative IOP control (Hilton, 1985; Jackson, 2000). As refinements in 20-gauge vitrectomy continued, smaller gauge systems were developed.

The initial description of small gauge vitrectomy, preceded its adoption by many years. The initial set of 25-gauge instruments developed by de Juan and Hickingobtham contained only a pneumatic vitrector, scissors, and a membrane removal instrument for use in pediatric eyes (De Juan & Hickingbotham, 1990). A 23-gauge vitrectomy probe was introduced in 1990 by Peyman, although its intended application was limited to vitreous and retinal biopsy (Peyman, 1990). Small gauge pars plana vitrectomy was popularized by Gildo Fujii who introduced a sutureless, transconjunctival, 25-gauge PPV system for use in a variety of surgical cases in 2002 (Fujii et al., 2002). Two years later, Dutch Ophthalmic Research Center (DORC) working with Klaus Eckardt presented the first 23-gauge vitrectomy system (Eckardt, 2005). Alcon laboratories subsequently developed a single step 23-gauge vitrectomy system. The exploration of yet smaller gauge instruments continued with the introduction of a 27-gauge vitrectomy system in 2010 by Oshima (Oshima et al. 2010).

Since the initial introduction, small-gauge vitrectomy has seen tremendous growth in popularity amongst retinal surgeons. According to the Preference and Trends (PAT) survey conducted annually by the American Society of Retina Specialists, 48% of its members who responeded in 2004 had never tried small-gauge vitrectomy. By 2007, however, 80% of respondents used it for certain surgical cases (Mittra & Pollak, 2007).

3. Preoperative considerations

As our experience with this new technology has increased, the clinical application of small gauge vitrectomy (27-, 25-, 23-gauge) has expanded tremendously over the past 10 years. This growth has been fueled by the development of a wide array of small gauge instruments produced by multiple manufacturers for the various vitrectomy systems.

3.1 Indications

The surgical scope for small gauge instruments was initially limited to less challenging cases such as epiretinal membrane removal and macular hole repair. With increased surgical experience, improved endoillumination, and development of a wide array of instruments, the use of small gauge vitrectomy has expanded to include nearly all surgical cases. Although specific considerations need to be made, small gauge surgery, both 25- and 23-gauge, can now be performed for complex cases including rhegmatogenous retinal detachments (RD), posteriorly subluxed lens extraction, tractional RD, RD with giant retinal tears, and combined vitrectomy and scleral buckle procedure. Tractional retinal detachments from diabetic retinopathy or proliferative vitreoretinopathy are now commonly performed using small gauge vitrectomy, and even considered to be ideal for these surgeries (Charles, 2007).

Silicion oil injection can now be performed using both 25- and 23- gauge instruments, most commonly with 1000 centistokes silicone oil (Erakgun & Egrilmez, 2009). Certain cases, such as removal of intraocular foreign body (IOFB), traumatic retinal detachment, biopsy of uveal melanoma, and vitreous or choroidal biopsy for intraocular lymphoma, that were initially felt to be feasible only with 20-gauge instruments, have now been performed successfully using small gauge systems (Abi-Ayed et al, 2011; Elrich & Franzco, 2011; Fabian & Moisseiev, 2011; Kunikata et al., 2011; Yeh et al, 2010; Trikha et al., 2010). Initial concerns that small gauge vitrectomy may lead to diminished sensitivity of vitreous biopsy for intraocular lymphoma do not appear to be supported by experimental data (Trikha et al,

2010). Most recently a 23-gauge combined endoscope, laser and illuminator has been developed for both vitrectomy and endolaser cyclophotocoagulation.

Small gauge vitrectomy offers a major advantage in pediatric surgeries, where close proximity of intraocular structures and reduced space for sclerotomy placement make larger gauge instruments more challenging to use (Gonzales, 2006, 2009). It has been successfully used in pediatric cases involving retinopathy of prematurity, vitreous hemorrhage, rhegmatogenous retinal detachment, persistent fetal vasculature, cataract, dislocated lens, endophthalmitis, macular pucker, traumatic macular hole, familial exudative vitreoretinopathy, and retained lens fragment (Gonzales, 2009). Hybrid vitrectomy techniques utilize both 20-gauge and small gauge ports, and can be employed when specific small gauge instrumentation is insufficient or not available (Kongsap, 2010). This technique can also be utilized to decrease surgical time when instilling or removing 5,000 centistoke silicone oil. Currently, small gauge pars plana lensectomy is only effecfive on soft cataracts, while dense cataracts require at least one 20-gauge port, although 23-gauge phacofragmenters are currently being developed (Thompson, 2011).

The table below lists some of the many indications for small gauge vitrectomy in both adult and pediatric eyes.

Adult	Pediatric
ERM Peel	ROP
Macular Hole	Vitreous hemorrhage
Posteriorly Subluxed Lens	Cataract extraction
Tractional RD	Endophthalmitis
Silicone Oil Injection	ERM Peel
Vitreous Hemorrhage	Macualar hole
Rhegatogenous RD	FEVR
Uveal/ Vitreous Biopsy	Persistent fetal vasculature
IOFB Removal	Retained lens fragments
Endophthalmitis	

Table 1. Indications for small gauge vitrectomy in adult and pediatric eyes.

3.2 Previous ocular surgery

Eyes that have undergone, or might undergo, a glaucoma filtering surgery are excellent candidates for small gauge surgery (Recchia et al., 2010). The small incisions created by 25- and 23-gauge vitrectomy, reduces conjunctival trauma and allows for preservation of filtering blebs. Additionally, eyes that have recent corneal or scleral wounds from surgery or trauma can develop wound leakage during trocar insertion. Wounds should be inspected and sutured if necessary prior to creating new incisions.

4. Small gauge vitrectomy design

The development of small gauge instrumentation has been fueled by the quest for decreased ocular truma, faster patient recovery, and shorter surgical time. These advantages have come with a few drawbacks specific to the gauge and design of the vitrectomy system, and the surgical techniques utilized. With decreasing size, there has been tremendous focus not only on the design of the vitrector, but also on illumination, laser, and multifunction instruments.

With small vitrectomy instruments, scleral incision size has significantly been reduced. Table 2 lists the sizes of the incisions created using the avaiable vitrecomy instruments. Prior to the use of small gauge instruments, PPV required conjunctival and scleral incisions, both of which needed suturing at the conclusion of the procedure. The use of small gauge vitrectomy instruments allows the surgeon to create a single, transconjunctival, scleral incision for access to the vitreous.

Gauge	Scleral Incision Size (mm)
19-G	1.1
20-G	0.9
23-G	0.60
25-G	0.50
27-G	0.40

Table 2. Scleral Incision Size Created by Various Guage Vitrectomy Systems

4.1 Trocar cannula system

Sutureless, transconjunctival 25-gauge vitrectomy was the first widely used small gauge vitrectomy system. Initially developed by Bausch & Lomb (B&L Rochester, NY) it was quickly adopted by other manufactures. The basic surgical technique is similar to its 20-gauge precursor, with 3 scleral incisions made to allow for placement of infusion and instrument cannulas. A number of manufactures have now developed small gauge vitrectomy systems including Alcon (Alcon, Ft Worth, TX, USA), Synergetics Inc. (O'Fallon, MO, USA), and Dutch Ophthalmic, USA (Kingston, NH, USA).

The key to small gauge instrumentation is the use of a trocar cannula system, which allows for the simultaneous creation of a small-gauge sclerotomy and insertion of a flexible polyamide cannula. The conjunctival incisions are made while the trocar-cannula is passed in a single transconjunctival scleral incision for all vitrectomy ports. Prior to the trocar incision, the conjunctiva is displaced using a cotton tip applicator or forceps, to intentionally misalign the scleral and conjunctival openings. This allows the conjunctiva to cover the sclerotomy after the cannula is removed. The cannula remains in place during surgery and aligns both the conjunctival and scleral incisions, to allow for easy insertion and withdrawal of instruments. Care should be taken not to tear the conjunctiva during displacement, especially when using forceps. Although conjunctival displacement is intended to reduce the risk of contamination of the scleral wound after surgery, it has not demonstrated prevention of ocular surface fluid from entering the scleral wound in experimental studies (Singh, A. et al., 2008).

The trocar cannula system is composed of a microcannula that is mounted onto a sharp trocar. Since the original development, the trocar cannula system has been modified with improvements in the trocar needle design and sharpness, allowing for improved wound construction and easier cannula placement. The cannula is composed of a polyamide tube mounted to a polymer cannula hub or collar. The cannula creates an entry port through the conjunctiva and sclera. The collar maintains the position of the cannula, and prevents it from sliding too far into the vitreous chamber. The collar also provides a platform to allow the surgeon to grasp the cannula, and some have an opening that is funnel-shaped to assist during instrument insertion.

Trocar cannula system includes plugs that can be fitted into the cannula collar to occlude the opening. The plug is designed with a tapered shaft that provides a tight fit into the cannula port. It is important not to force the plug too deep within the cannula to avoid difficulty during removal. During removal it is helpful to have a second instrument to stabilizing the cannula hub during removal. This will help inadvertent withdrawal of the entire cannula if the plug is tightly fitted. Additionally, if there is forceful egress of fluid from an open cannula, lowering of the IOP will reduce the risk of projectile plug expulsion due to high outflow pressure from the port. The infusion is a metallic tube that is designed to fit into a cannula port. The cannula system has the added advantage of interchangeability of the instrument and infusion sites, which allows for improved access in certain cases. Valved cannulas have been introduced for obviate the need to cannula plugs when the port is not being utilized. This can reduce the risk of intraoperative hypotony, but also increases the possibility of accidental cannula removal when withdrawing an instrument due to increased friction from the cannula valves on the instrument.

4.2 Wound construction

In standard 20-gauge vitrectomy surgery, conjunctival incisions are made to expose the sclera in preparation for sclerotomy placement. A microvitreoretinal blade (MVR) is used to make perpendicular incisions through the sclera, 3 to 4 mm posterior to the limbus. The infusion cannula is placed in the inferotemporal region, and sutured to the sclera to avoid accidental dislocation intraoperatively. Two additional sclerotomies are made near the 10 and 2 o'clock positions for instrument access to the vitreous cavity. Although 20-gauge cannulas are available and used by some, vitrectomy instruments in 20-gauge vitrectomy are most commonly passed directly through the scleral incisions without the use of a cannula system (Rizzo et al., 2009).

The most critical step in small gauge vitrectomy is the configuration and correct placement of the scleral incisions. The early descriptions of small gauge sclerotomies involved creating a perpendicular transconjunctival incision with conjunctival displacement (Fujii et al., 2002). This technique was modified to an oblique scleral incision after studies demonstrated better wound closure and reduced risk of hypotony (Hsu et al., 2008; Inoue et al., 2007; Taban et al., 2009). R.P. Singh et al. in a histopathologic study using rabbit eyes demonstrated increased leakage of intraocular dye in straight (perpendicular) incisions versus angled (oblique) incisions, in both 25- and 23-gauge vitrectomy systems (R.P. Singh et al., 2008). Similarly, Gupta et al., demonstrated decreased wound integrity in eyes that underwent 25-gauge PPV with perpendicular scleral incisions compared to beveled incision (Gupta et al., 2009). In this study, dye placed on the ocular surface of human cadaver eyes had more wound penetration in 25-gauge perpendicular incisions then in 25-gauge beveled incisions. Taban et al., utilizing both optical coherence tomography and india ink ingress, evaluated differences in wound integrity with both 25- and 23-gauge, straight and angled incisions on cadaver eyes (Taban et al., 2008). This study found that angled incisions had better wound apposition under dynamic IOP than stright incisions. India ink applied to the surface after incisions were made fully penetrated through some straight incisions, but were not found in any of the angled wounds.

Shelved sclerotomy construction has been described in a one-step or two-step method. The one-step incision involves simultaneous entry of a sharp trochar with a mounted cannula. The trocar is removed and the cannula left in place for the remainder of the surgery. One-step oblique incisions can be made perpendicular or parallel to the limbus (Lopez-Guajardo et al., 2006, Shimada et al. 2006). Due to the orientation of scleral fibers in this region, scleral incisions made parallel to the limbus offers a theoretical benefit of displacing scleral fibers, rather than cutting them, as in incisions that are perpendicular to the limbus (Lopez-Guajardo et al., 2006). In addition, incisions that run parallel to the limbus are less likely to encroach the lens or retina.

Additional modifications to the one-step incisions have been made to improve wound architecture. A biplanar scleral incision involves changing the angle of entry during insertion of the trocar blade through the sclera. One variation includes initiating the scleral incision at a 30-degree angle tangential to the sclera, then repositioning to an angle that is perpendicular once the blade has partially entered the sclera. Alternatively, a more acute (5 degree) initial entry angle can be made with a more vertical angle upon completion of the scleral tunnel. Although no clinical trial we could find demonstrated a significant benefit of this biplanar scleral incision, it does offer the benefit of avoiding the peripheral retina after the trocar has entered the vitreous.

In the two-step method, the displaced conjunctiva is stabilized with a pressure plate instrument, while a shelved incision is created using a sharp angled blade (Eckardt, 2005). The blade is removed and a cannula is inserted along the same transconjunctival path using a blunt trocar. Advantages of the two-step method, including more consistent wound creation and improved stabilization of the eye with the pressure plate, are off set by the increased difficulty in spate placement of the cannula as well as increased overall time. Correct location for sclerotomy placement can be determined by using traditional calipers, or by using the fixed caliper that is now found on most small gauge vitrectomy systems. Trocar fixed calipers cause minimal conjunctival trauma, and allow the surgeon to quickly measure between 3 and 4 mm from the corneal limbus, eliminating the need for an additional instrument.

Due to the reduced caliber of small gauge vitrectomy instruments, flexion of the instruments during manipulation of the globe, poses a major disadvantage. For this reason, in small gauge vitrectomy, the location of the superior vitrectomy ports should be made as close as possible to the horizontal plane of the eye (Figure 1). This reduces the need to rotate the instruments significantly to access the peripheral and superior retina. By limiting the torsion placed on the globe, there is less distortion of the scleral wound, and reduced issues with tool flexion. The superonasal trocar entry should be placed in a location that would allow the least restriction by the bridge of the nose during surgery. The superotemporal trocar entry should be made near the horizontal plane of the eye, in the area corresponding to the lowest point of the supraorbital rim (Charles et al, 2007). The infusion is usually placed in the inferotemporal location, and can easily be transferred during surgery to either of the other cannulas.

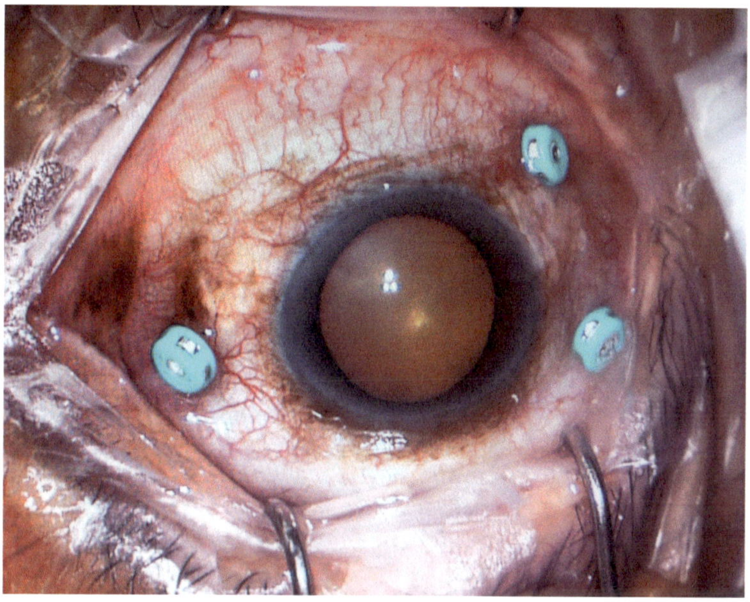

Fig. 1. Transconjunctival 25-Gauge vitrectomy ports placed in right eye. Note the trocars are valved to avoid fluid egress. The superior sclerotomy sites are seen at the bottom of the image. The upper right port in the image is the infusion site, and is located in the inferotemporal quadrant of the globe.

4.3 Fluidics

Vitreous has physical properties of both a solid and a liquid. It is 98% water, with the remaining material composed mostly of a matrix of collagen fibrils, large molecules of hyaluronic acid, non-collagenous proteins, glycoproteins, salts and sugars. Because of its dual liquid and solid physical properties, and attachment to intraocular structures, vitreous has to be excised as it is removed to reduce traction on the retina. This requirement necessitated the need for the development of the current vitrectomy instrument. Understanding of the flow of vitreous and liquid though the various vitrectomy systems has important clinical relevance.

The flow of a non-compressible fluid through a tube is governed by Poiseuille's equation. Based on this formula, the flow rate is directly proportional to the inner radius of the tube to the fourth power, and the pressure gradient on either end. Flow rate is inversely related to the length of the tube and the viscosity of the fluid. The clinical application of this principle to small gauge vitrectomy shows that the inner diameter of the small gauge vitrectomy systems will have the greatest impact on the flow of fluid, into and out of the eye. Studies, however, have shown that since the vitreous does not behave as liquid, other factors affecting flow, including vacuum pressure, cut rate and duty cycle of the vitrector are critical features governing flow rate in clinical settings (Hubschman et al 2008; Magalhaes et al. 2009). Fujii et al., in their introduction of a 25-gauge vitrectomy system reported a 40% greater flow rate with 25-gauge vitrectomy at 1500 cuts per minute (cpm) and 500 mmHg of vacuum, compared to 20-gauge vitrectomy at 750 cpm and 250 mmHg of vacuum (Fujii et al., 2002). They went on to report, however, that flow rates with 25-gauge (at 500 mmHg vacuum and 1500 cpm) was 2.3 times lower then 20-gauge vitrectomy at a high cut rate (250 mmHg vacuum and 1500 cpm).

The basic principle of the vitrector is to create a suction force into the port, allowing for vitreous to enter, and then cutting this segment of vitreous to relieve traction on the remaining vitreous body. The duty cycle in this process refers to the percentage of time the cutter port is open relative to each cutting cycle. Duty cycle varies depending on the type of vitrectomy drive mechanism utilized (Magalhaes et al., 2009). The three major types of drive mechanisms for vitrectomy handpieces are the guillotine electric, guillotine pneumatic, and the reciprocating rotary pneumatic. The electric drive system maintains a constant duty cycle regardless of cutting speed. The guillotine pneumatic drive system produces a high duty cycle (port is open longer than it is closed during each cycle) during slow cut rates, and a low duty cycle at high cut rates (port is closed longer than it is open). Finally, the reciprocating rotary pneumatic cutter also provides a constant duty cycle regardless of cut rate (Rizzo et al., 2009). In the guillotine pneumatic cutter, variation in duty cycle occurs because the speed at which the cutter closes is faster than the speed at which the cutter opens. The opening speed in this system is limited by relatively slower spring mechanism employed to place the cutter back into its open port position. During high cut rates, the inability of the spring drive opening to keep up with the pneumatically driven closure, increases the time the port is in the closed position, thereby decreasing the duty cycle. In the reciprocating pneumatic cutter, a duel line system is utilized, allowing for port closure and opening to be pneumatically driven at the same rates. The newest pneumatic vitrectomy systems employ this technology and allow the surgeon to vary duty cycle between 50% (the port is open and closed for the same duration in a cut cycle, similar to electric drive cutters), less than 50% (biased towards closed port), or more than 50% (biased towards open port) (Alcon Constellation® and Bausch & Lomb Stellaris PC®). Since the optimal duty cycle varies depending on the physical properties of the material being removed, some believe pneumatic vitreous cutters are more versatile during vitreo-retinal surgery (Charles et al, 2007).

Cut rates of all vitrectomy systems have increased since the original design. This movement has been propelled by the belief that higher cut rates will decrease vitreous traction during all aspects of vitrectomy. High cut rates have traditionally come at the cost of reduced flow and removal of vitreous. This effect of cut rate on flow was seen with the older generation pneumatic cutters in the leading vitrectomy system (Accurus®), but was not seen in electric vitrectomy cutters. The latest vitrectomy systems are capable of cut rates up to 5000 cpm in 20-, 23-, and 25-gauge formats (Constellation® and Stellaris PC®). These vitrectomy systems both employ duel line pneumatic cutters that allow for 50% duty cycle at the highest cut rates.

4.4 Infusion

Small gauge vitrectomy systems utilize a cannula-based infusion line that has a precise sliding fit within the microcannula. The fit is tight enough to provide enough resistance to prevent ejection under high infusion pressures. Balanced salt solution (BSS) flow rate through the infusion cannula is most influenced by the diameter of the lumen of the tube and microcannula (Rizzo et al, 2009).

4.5 Vitreous cutter design

The general design of the vitreous cutters in micorincisional surgery is the same as 20-gauge vitreous cutters. Electric vitrectors are much larger in overall size then pneumatic cutters, regardless of the gauge used. The major differences between newly designed small gauge vitrectomy probes and traditional 20-gauge vitrectomy probes, are lumen diameter, stiffness of the shaft and distance of the vitrectomy port from end of the probe.

Stiffness of the vitrectomy probe becomes clinically relevant in surgery that requires significant eye rotation to reach peripheral retina. Hubschman et al., studied the stiffness of 25-, 23-, and 20-gauge vitrectomy probes from various developers (Hubschman et al., 2008). Stiffness of the shaft of each vitrectomy probe was determined by measuring the displacement of the tip of the probe under a constant force. The study found that differences in probe stiffness was explained by differences in metal properties, thickness in shaft wall (difference between external and internal diameter), and probe length.

The external and internal diameters of the various probes were also measured. There was very little variation in the external diameter among the four 25-gauge probes (0.5mm) and two 23-gauge probes (0.5mm) (Hubschman et al, 2008). This is to be expected, since the gauge of vitrectomy instruments is classified based on the external diameter. Interestingly, the internal diameter varied significantly among 25-gauge (range 227 um to 292 um) and 23-gauge (355 um to 318 um) vitrectomy probes.

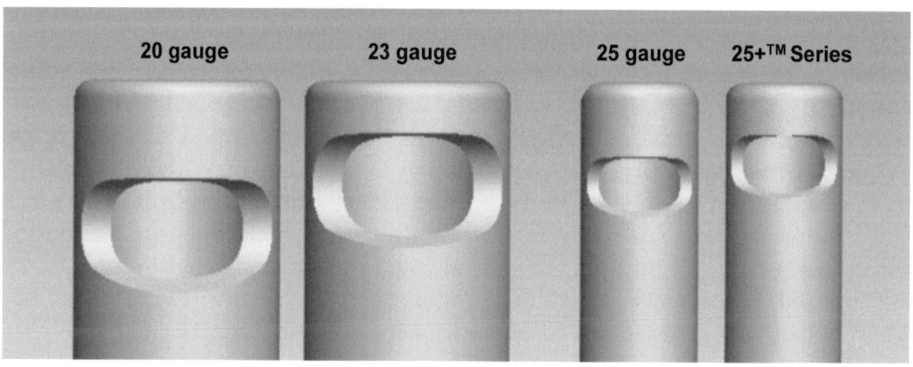

Fig. 2. Vitrectomy probes of various gauge systems (Alcon, Ft Worth, TX, USA). Note the port opening size and location. The port opening location is closer to the the end of the probe in both the 23-gauge and 25-gauge systems compared to the conventional 20-gauge system.

Another major advantage in design of small gauge vitrectomy has been the displacement of the opening closer to the end of the vitrectomy probe. This shift has been made possible by increased vitrectomy cut rates and improvements in fluids of the vitrectomy systems, both of which have made it safer to operate closer to the retina. Although delamination and segmentation using intraocular scissors is still necessary in many cases, positioning of the port closer to the probe tip has made it possible to dissect epiretinal membranes using the vitrector alone. This has proven to be of great value removing preretinal membranes in patients with proliferative diabetic retinopathy.

4.6 Endoillumination

Smaller gauge endoillumination probes initially produced significantly reduced light output compared to the 20-gauge probes. The development of higher-output light sources and wide-angle light probes has eliminated inadequate illumination in small gauge vitrectomy. Although, brighter light can be achieved with new xenon and mercury vapor sources, the risk of phototoxicity should be considered, especially during macular surgery. Illuminated infusion cannulas and chandelier lights are also available and allow for bimanual surgery. Improved quality of illuminated laser probes enables more efficient delivery of laser, along with the option for surgeon-performed depressed exam and peripheral laser.

A Chandelier light is now available in 25- and 27-gauge light probes, and is inserted in the pars plana to provide a continuous, hands-free illumination of the vitreous cavity. This light probe is usually placed inferiorly, although it can be inserted elsewhere depending on surgeon's need and preference. Directing the chandelier probe more posteriorly than the usual entry angle reduces glare and allows for diffuse endoillumination of the posterior chamber (Charles et al, 2007). Although the use of this device allows for true bimanual surgery, it has limited utility compared conventional light probes.

4.7 Cannula withdrawal and wound closure

At the completion of the surgery, the cannulas are removed using forceps, with simultaneous application of pressure on the scleral wound using a cotton tip applicator. If a valved cannula is not being used, instrument ports should be closed with a plug at the time of the cannula removal. This allows for inspection of the wound for leakage, and suturing if necessary. Just prior to removal of a cannula, the infusion is clamped or the pressure is lowered to 5 mmHg. With pressure applied to the scleral wound using a cotton tip applicator, the infusion is activated to a pressure of 25 to 30 mmHg. With this technique, the internal pressure from the infusion and the external pressure from the cotton tip forces the shelved incision to close. The conjunctiva is gently pushed back to its original position to cover the sclerotomy. The infusion is removed last, as with standard vitrectomy. If wound leakage is noted, a dissolvable suture is placed through the conjunctiva and sclera to close the sclerotomy. In some situations, chemosis or hemorrhage reduces the ability to visualize the scleral wound, and a small conjunctival incision is necessary for suture placement. If the eye is hypotonus after removal of all cannulas, then BSS or sterile air is injected to achieve optimal IOP. Some surgeons perform a partial air-fluid exchange at the completion of surgery to reduces risk of hypotony. The increased surface tension of air versus liquid is felt to reduce the wound leakage from the sclerotomy sites.

5. Surgical technique

The general procedure for small gauge vitrectomy is the same as with traditional 20-gauge vitrectomy. Standard sterile procedure using povidone-iodine (Betadine 5%) is utilized to prepare the eye, and instilled on the ocular surface. Sterile drapes are used per standard protocol. In small gauge vitrectomy, the use of an adjustable lid speculum is advantageous over spring retractors. This mostly relates to the ability to reduce lid retraction to provide increased conjunctival laxity for sufficient displacement during trocar insertion.

Disposable trocars for small gauge surgery come pre-loaded with cannulas. Care should be taken by the assistant to avoid inadvertent removal and loss of the cannula during handling. Measurements are made for sclerotomy location, and can be done using fixed calipers on the back of the trocar, if present. Most surgeons place cannulas 3.0 mm to 3.5 mm posterior to the limbus in aphakic or pseudophakic eyes, and 3.5 to 4.0 mm in phakic eyes. A cotton-tipped swab is best for displacing the conjunctiva since it is least traumatic, and less likely to create a tear that would require suturing. The scleral mark created from the caliper should be visible through the displaced conjunctiva. The trocar is inserted in an oblique angle, parallel to the limbus, and oriented more vertically prior to entering the vitreous. The 23-gauge cannulas should to be inserted at a more acute angle (5 degrees) then 25- or 27-gauge systems. This allows for a longer scleral tunnel and better wound closure. With this method a two-step incision reduces the risk of penetration into peripheral pars plana after entry into the vitreous.

The infusion port is placed first, usually in the inferotemporal region. Sterile drape or tape is used to secure the infusion line and direct it to the mid-vitreous. Correct positioning of the cannula in the vitreous is verified prior to infusion activation. The superior cannulas are then inserted near the 10 and 2 o'clock positions. As mentioned earlier, with smaller gauge systems, positioning of the superior cannulas closer to the horizontal plane of the eye improves access to the superior peripheral retina. The instruments can then be inserted for vitrectomy. When removing instruments, the cannula should be observed for inadvertent removal. If the cannula appears loose, then forceps should be utilized during instrument removal. If the cannula is accidentally removed, it can be reloaded onto the trocar and inserted into the same wound if possible. Otherwise, a new transconjunctival incision is made in a new location.

5.1 Macular surgery

Macular surgery is an ideal indication for small gauge vitrectomy, as it requires less manipulation of the instruments and less need for thorough dissection of the peripheral retina. Indications for this surgery include macular pucker, macular hole, vitreomacular traction syndrome, macular edema, subhyaloid or submacular hemorrhage. As with most vitrectomy surgeries, a core vitrectomy is first performed. This is usually followed by induction of a posterior vitreous detachment (PVD), if not already present. This step highlights a disadvantage in some of the small gauge vitrectomy systems, where substantially low flow rates create difficulty in detaching the vitreous from the optic nerve. The vitreous cutter or a soft tip cannula can be utilized, and is set to active extrusion between 400 and 500 mmHg. The infusion rate should be increased if hypotony is noted during active suction. The soft-tip cannula or vitrector is held at the disc margin and aspiration is applied. The cutter should be turned off if using the vitrector. Engagement of adherent vitreous is seen as a slight elevation of the disc margin due to vitreous traction. Anterior movement of the aspiration instrument is often sufficient to detach the vitreous from the nerve, but in some cases, tangential traction is also required to achieve this result. Vitreous staining can be done using triamcinolone and can identify any residual adherent vitreous. If the posterior hyaloid is strongly adherent, a bent MVR blade or a long 25-gauge needle can be used to separate the posterior hyaloid around the optic nerve. This is best performed using a contact lens for improved visualization. Once separated form the optic nerve, the vitrector or soft-tip can be used to elevate the hyaloid over the macula. Extra care should to be employed in diabetic patients to avoid trauma to adherent blood vessels.

If epiretinal membrane (ERM) or internal limiting membrane (ILM) peeling is necessary a macular contact lens is utilized. Some surgeons prefer to create a membrane edge using micro-pick, bent MVR blade or needle, or a diamond dusted membrane scraper. Once an edge has been created, membrane forceps can be used to carefully strip the tissue from the retinal surface. For peeling of the ERM or ILM, staining of the retina can be performed using indocyanine green (ICG), trypan blue, or triamcinolone. Use of these agents can also uncover incomplete vitreous separation from the posterior pole. Additionally, use of stains can help ensure complete peeling of the ILM and ERM of the central macular region, and possibly reduce the risk of reoperation. This benefit must be weighed against the potential risk of ocular toxicity that has been suspected with the use of some of these dyes (Rodrigues, EB et al., 2007).

Removal of membranes from the retinal surface using 25-gauge instruments can occasionally result in paradoxical movement of the tip of the forceps. This occurs because of flexion forces near the proximal end of the forceps create a reverse movement of the distal end of the forceps, in attempted rotation of the eye. If this occurs during membrane peeling, repositioning of the forceps and engaging a different area of the membrane to avoid tension on the globe will eliminate the problem. The increased stiffness of 23-gauge and newer 25-gauge instruments has nearly eliminated this effect.

Treatment for submacular hemorrhage can be performed by injection of subretinal tissue plasminogen activator (TPA). This technique can be performed with the use of any of the small gauge vitrectomy systems. A subretinal cannula, such as a 39-gauge submacular cannula is connected to a 3 ml syringe via extension tubing. TPA is used off label at a concentration of 12 ug/ 0.1 ml. Standard vitrectomy with PVD induction is performed. The subretinal cannula is then inserted directly through the retina without the need for a retinotomy. Injection using this technique should be performed over an area of subretinal hemorrhage, so that displacement of the subretinal hemorrhage can provide a visual clue that would indicate entry through the retina. Sufficient TPA is injected to create retinal elevation in the macula. Some surgeons use perfluorocarbon liquid to displace the liquefied hemorrhage away from the central macula, but this is not required. Laser photocoagulation is not required to seal the entry site of the submacular cannula. A peripheral retinal exam is performed as with all vitrectomy surgery, followed by air-fluid exchange and gas instillation. The choice of gas in this setting is surgeon dependent, but a short acting gas is sufficient to allow for displacement of subretinal hemorrhage. The patient is instructed to remain upright postoperatively for up to 1 week to allow for displacement of the hemorrhage.

5.2 Diabetic retinopathy

Surgical indications for diabetic retinopathy include non-clearing vitreous hemorrhage (VH), tractional retinal detachment (TRD), refractory diabetic macular edema, premacular subhyaloid hemorrhage, and ghost-cell glaucoma. With the expansion of small gauge surgical tools, 25- and 23- gauge vitrectomy cannot only be utilized for nearly all cases, but also offers a few additional advantages.

The surgical approach to performing ERM or ILM peeling, and relieving vitreomacular traction in diabetic patients are the same as in 20-gauge procedures. Special considerations for performing PVD and membrane peeling using small gauge systems have been discussed earlier. For treatment of VH and TRD, the main goals are to clear the media and relieve macular traction. Eyes with a complete PVD preoperative are less likely to need vitrectomy, due to the lack of hyaloidal traction on the retina. Non-clearing vitreous hemorrhags are easily cleared with 23- and 25-gauge systems, and are more recently being performed with 27-gauge vitrectomy. The initial limiting factor of reduced flow and increased vitrectomy time with small gauge vitrectors has become less important with improvement in system fluidics. Endolaser probes are available in a variety of styles, including fixed curved and extendable cuved, which allow for excellent access to peripheral retina without the need for significant rotation of the eye.

Diabetic tractional retinal detachments are treated with three basic surgical approaches. After performing a core vitrectomy and relieving anterior-posterior vitreous traction where possible, dissection of the posterior hyaloid from retinal adhesions is performed using the following techinques: segmentation, delamination, or en bloc separation. Segmentation involves severing vitreous adhesions between focal points of retinal attachments, leaving isolated segments of fibrovascular tissue adherent to the retina, without vitreo-retinal traction. Delamination, in contrast, involves separation of all vitreo-retinal attachments by dissecting parallel to the plane of the retina, with no residual fibrovascular tissue on the retinal surface. En bloc dissection involves separating the vitreous body and all adherent fibrovascular membranes as a single unit (Charles et al., 2007; Rizzo et al., 2009).

The size of the small gauge vitreous cutters and the more distal location of the vitrectomy port offer an advantage when performing dissection of fibrovascular tissue near the retina. The vitreous cutter can be used as a scissor to cut fibrous tissue with little traction on the retina. This reduces the need and frequency of repeatedly inserting vertical or horizontal scissors, although these are available in a variety of small gauge options. The added stiffness of 25 and 23-gauge instruments, along with the options for small gauge silicone oil instillation leaves very few diabetic vitrectomies that require large gauge instruments.

Ghost-cell glaucoma represents a complication of dense, chronic vitreous hemorrhage, with migration of degenerated red blood cells into the anterior chamber, and blockage of the trabecular meshwork with red blood cell debris or macrophages. Vitrectomy is performed in the setting of uncontrolled IOP, despite medical treatment. Small gauge vitrectomy systems allow for easy access of the vitrector, or even the infusion, into the anterior chamber through a paracentesis.

5.3 Rhegmatogenous retinal detachment

For uncomplicated rhegamatogenous RD, pars plana vitrectomy has become more widely used as a primary treatment technique, especially for pseudophakic and aphakic eyes. Benefits for vitrectomy over scleral buckling include controlled drainage of subretinal fluid, ability to remove vitreous opacities, identification of small breaks, minimal or no effect on refractive error. Vitrectomy, especially small gauge systems, causes less trauma to conjunctiva and sclera, avoids muscle manipulation, allows control of intraoperative pressure, and causes less patient discomfort after surgery, although this has not been proven. The increased incidence of cataract formation with vitrectomy is well known, and should be considered when selecting the surgical option. The risk for increased proliferative vitreoretinopathy (PVR) with vitrectomy compared to scleral buckling has not been proven, but is a debated issue.

Techniques for repair of rhegamatogenous retinal detachments using small gauge vitrectomy are similar to those using 20-gauge systems. Infusion pressures and aspiration for 25-gauge are set higher than those for 20-gauge vitrectomy, usually in the range of 35 to 45 mmHg for infusion, and between 600 mmHg for aspiration during vitrectomy. Superior ports should be placed close to the horizontal meridian to allow for increased access to the superior peripheral retina. A chandelier light infusion can be used but ais usually not necessary. A variety of techniques are available to repair the retinal detachment depending on surgeon preference. A lighted laser allows the surgeon to perform scleral depression and simultaneously apply laser. Gas is most commonly used as a tamponade agent. For gas exchange, typically the surgeon removes one superior cannula and instills the gas mixture through the infusion cannula, although other techniques are also available. When using small gauge surgery, it is important to save some of the gas mixture until all cannulas are removed and inspected for leaks. If a sclerotomy demonstrates leakage and needs to be sutured, then the appropriate gas mixture can be injected upon completion to attain optimal IOP.

Silicone oil can now be injected and extracted using an automated system with both 23- and 25-gauge ports. Injecting high viscosity silocone oil (5000 cs) is very time consuming with this approach and does not offer any proven benefits over lower viscosity oil (1000 cs). Oil injection is performed in the same fashion as in 20-gauge vitrectomy, using very low infusion pressures. In combined scleral bucke and vitrectomy procedures, many surgeons use standard 20-gauge vitrectomy since the conjunctival incisions have to be made. Using a small gauge system with combined scleral buckle cases, however, does offer some benefits. For this procedure, a 360-degree conjunctival peritomy is made with isolation of the recti muscles using 2-0 silk ties. All buckle components can then be placed prior to vitrectomy. If the preference is to tie scleral sutures after vitrectomy, the infusion cannula can be temporarily relocated to a superior port to allow for better access to the inferotemporal quadrant. Scleral incisions using the trocar can still be made in a shelved fashion, and be left sutureless if no leak is seen.

5.4 Pars plana lensectomy

Small gauge vitrectomy is a viable alternative to the standard 20-gauge vitrectomy with phacofragmentation for retained lens fragments after complicated cataract surgery. In 2008, Kiss and Vavvas reported successful use of 25-gauge vitrectomy for the removal of retained crystalline lens (Kiss & Vavvas, 2008). In this study, they found that the 25-gauge vitreous cutter allowed for removal of softer lens material, however, cases involving dense nuclear fragments required sclerotomy enlargement and use of the 20-gauge phacofragmatome (Kiss & Vavvas, 2008). Similarly, Laurence Ho et al. also reported successful outcomes using 25-gauge vitrectomy to remove retained lens fragments (Ho, 2010). Removal of the vitreous surrounding the lens fragment is performed from anterior to posterior. After a compete vitrectomy with removal of all vitreous traction on the lens, the cutter can be set to a reduced speed, as low as 600 cpm, to remove lens material. The light pipe can be used to break up large lens fragments at the vitrectomy probe. The final visual outcomes for small gauge lensectomy have been reported to be similar to those obtained using the 20-gauge vitrectomy system. Incidence of postoperative complications after 25-gauge vitrectomy for retained lens fragments including glaucoma, cystoid macular edema and retinal detachment, was similar to that seen with 20-gauge instrumentation (Ho, 2010).

5.5 Pediatric surgery

Small gauge vitrectomy has been utilized for a wide variety of vitreoretinal disorders in the pediatric population. A major concern for the use of this technology for patients in this age group is the risk of hypotony and it associated complications. Children are more likely to rub their eyes and thus may cause wound leakage in the immediate postoperative period. Hypotony in children with vasoproilferative disorders could result in bleeding from sensitive vascular tissue. Sclerotomies in young children are made in the pars plicata, just posterior to the limbus, so sufficient conjunctival displacement of the sclerotomy incisions is difficult. To improve saftey, some surgeons advocate suturing of both sclera and conjunctiva in younger childern undergoing small gauge vitrectomy (Gonzales et al, 2006). Potential advantages that have been suggested with the use of small gauge vitrectomy in this subset of patients include increased accessibility to smaller spaces within the eye, such as between the lens and ridges in patients with retinopathy of prematurity (ROP), or between tight retinal folds in cases of tractional RD (Gonzales et al, 2009). Additionally, due to the small size of the eye and immature pars plana, small gauge vitrectomy allows for the use of 3 ports in some pediatric eyes that would otherwise have room for only two, 20-gauge ports.

Gonzales et al., reported successful outcomes for small gauge vitrectomy in pediatric eyes involving tractional RD secondary to retinopathy of prematurity (ROP), vitreous hemorrhage, rhegmatogenous RD, familial exudative vitreoretinopathy (FEVR), persistent fetal vasculature, cataract, dislocated lens, macular pucker, endophthalmitis, exudative RD, traumatic macular hole, retained lens material and aqueous misdirection (Gonzales et al., 2009). In their report, however, the authors cautioned that 25-gauge vitrectomy may not be the best approach in all pediatric surgery. It is possible that some limitations experienced with 25-gauge insturments, specifically, instrument stiffness, could be overcome with 23-gauge systems.

5.5.1 Retinopathy of prematurity

Previously, retinal detachment due to ROP was repaired with scleral buckle, using PPV only when the sclera buckle failed. More recently however, PPV has been used as the primary surgical approach, thus allowing for direct removal of vitreous traction, decreased compression of the anterior ocular structures and less surgically induced myopia. Prior to the popularization of small gauge vitrectomy, 20-gauge vitrectomy was used for RD repair in these patients. In 2006, Gonzales et al., described the three-port, pars plicata vitrectomy technique for RD repair (Gonzales et al., 2006). Conjunctival dissection is performed followed by creation of sclerotomies 0.5 mm to 1.0 mm posterior to the limbus, in the pars plicata. The infusion line is placed inferotemporally, unless this is the site of the tractional RD. In that event, the infusion should be placed away from the RD. An MVR blade is used to make the sclerotomies in the superotemporal and superonasal quadrants; trocar cannula system is not used for this technique. Lens sparing vitrectomies are employed unless there is significant retinal-lental touch or lens opacities obscuring view to the posterior pole. Upon completion of the surgery, the conjunctival and scleral wounds are sutured. This technique is best utilized in cases where views to the posterior are clear, particularly when there are no anterior tractional retinal folds in close approximation to the lens or extensive anterior fibrosis. Hemorrhage, presence of plus disease, and neovascularization have been associated with poor surgical outcomes in repair of retinal detachment secondary to ROP (Gonzales et al., 2006).

6. Advantages of small gauge vitrectomy

Numerous advantages have been proposed for small gauge vitrectomy including decreased ocular trauma and inflammation, reduced conjunctival scaring, shorter operative time, increased patient comfort, and faster visual recovery.

6.1 Decreased ocular trauma

The reduced trauma from smaller conjunctival and scleral incisions made in 25-, 23- ,and 27-gauge surgeries has the theoretical advantages of reducing conjunctival scaring. This is of major importance in patients with previous or planned glaucoma surgery. In our experience it also limits irregular scar formation and conjunctival disfigurement.

6.2 Reduced surgical time

Fujii et al., in their initial report on 25-gauge vitrectomy, reported shorter operative times with sutureless vitrectomy compared to 20-gauge. Although they found slightly longer vitrectomy times due to reduced flow with the 25-gauge system, this was minimal in comparison to the time saved during opening and closing of the surgical wounds (Fujii et al., 2002). Reduced surgical times with small gauge sutureless vitrectomy has also been reported by others (Rizzo et al., 2006; Kadonosono et al., 2006). Some studies have shown, however, that the time saved in managing the incisions, was lost because of longer duration of vitrectomy, resulting in no significant difference in surgical time (Kellner et al., 2007; Wimpissingwer et al., 2008, as cited in Thompson, 2011). Although reduced time managing the surgical wound as been attributed to the reduced time for surgery, other factors including less vitreous removal and easier case selection also favor this finding.

6.3 Patient comfort and recovery

One of the major advantages of small gauge surgery is reduced postoperative pain (Mentens et al., 2009). small incision, as well as the lack of sclera and conjunctival sutures, are likely the major factors contributing to this finding. Additionally, visual recovery has been shown to be faster with small gauge vitrectomy, likely due to the lack of suture induced astigmatism found in 20-gauge vitrectomy (Hass et al., 2010). Patients in our practice rarely require narcotic medications for pain control following small gauge surgery, which were needed routinely following 20-gauge vitrectomy.

7. Complications of small gauge vitrectomy

7.1 Intraoperative

A number of intraoperative complications can occur with the use of small gauge vitrectomy systems. Most of these are related to the issue of IOP control, but also include suprachoroidal hemorrhage, retinal tears, and retinal toxicity from subconjunctival medications.

7.1.1 Hypotony

There is an increased risk of hypotony in small gauge PPV during the placement of the trocars. The force required to insert the trocar cannula complex is substantially greater than that required to insert the 20-gauge MVR blade. This additional force is ncessary because the trocars in small gauge surgery are not as sharp as 20-gauge MVR blades, and because the cannula is intended to be forced throught the slightly smaller trocar incision. The tight fit of the cannula in the scleral incision creates resistence to dislocation of the cannula during removal of instruments. Additionally, placement of trocars requires the application of a compressive force to the globe to penetrate the sclera at an oblique angle (Wu et al., 2011). This force on the globe during insertion of the trocars has been shown to increase the IOP to as high as 63.7 mmHg (Dalma-Weiszhausz et al., 2008). The redesign of some trocar needles has partially reduced this problem. In patients with recent corneal or scleral wounds, such as those with recent cataract surgery, penetrating keratoplasty, or repair of a ruptured globe, the initial trocar insertion can cause wound leak with resultant hypotony and its associated risks (Wong et al., 2010). Careful inspection of all ocular wounds should be made prior to placement of new surgical incisions. All suspicious wounds should be sutured prior to placement of vitrectomy ports.

Eyes that have undergone previous vitrectomy are also more likely to have hypotony during trochar placement. This is most evident during placement of the superior cannulas, following successful placement of the infusion cannula. As the superior cannula is being inserted, IOP elevation causes fluid from the vitreous cavity to be displaced into the infusion cannula, with resultant deformation of the globe. In non-vitrectomized eye, fluid egress through the infusion is restricted by vitreous plugging of the infusion port, thereby providing more resistance to compression. This issue can be addressed by temporally increasing infusion pressure at the time of trochar insertion for the second and third cannulas. Similarly, some surgeons do not always place a plug in the instrument cannula when inserting the final trochar, relying on the vitreous to temporarily plug the open cannula. Although this does not usually create an issue, eyes that have significantly liquefied vitreous or prior vitrectomy, have an increased risk of hypotony because intraocular fluid can easily escape from the open cannula.

7.1.2 Cannula related complications

The infusion is the source of a few complications during small gauge vitrectomy. First, the infusion cannula is not sutured to the sclera, therefore, it can inadvertently be dislocated or pulled out. This is most likey to occur during scleral depression. Sudden loss of infusion and resultant hypotony during surgery has its obvious complications, including hemorrhage, choroidal detachment and retinal trauma from intraocular instruments. The best immediate solution is to replace the infusion into any cannula to pressurize the globe. The dislocated cannula can then be placed over a trocar and reinserted.

The use of cannulas for instrumentation also has a direct effect on the infusion. In small gauge vitrectomy, high velocity flow from the infusion can occur if there is rapid removal of fluid from the eye through an open cannula during exchange of instruments. The high infusion pressure can cause direct mechanical trauma to the retina, increased dehydration if air-fluid exchange has already been performed, or high flow infusion into a macular hole with resultant injury. Valved cannulas have recently been released to address this issue. Unusual complications with small gauge instruments have also been reported including breakage and intraocular dislocatoin of a segment of a cannula tip, as well as intraocular breakage of the vitrectomy tip (Chen C. et al., 2008; Inoue et al., 2004).

7.2 Postoperative complications

7.2.1 Hypotony

Since the initial introduction of small gauge, sutureless vitrectomy, there has been a great deal of concern for postoperative hypotony. Several papers have reported the incidence of hypotony after 25-gauge vitrectomy, ranging from 3.8% to 16% (Chen E., 2007; Byeon, 2006). The wide range of incidence has mostly been attributed to variations in the definition of hypotony, incision technique, instrument design, variation in surgical manipulation of instruments, and surgical techniques (Chen D. et al., 2010). Hypotony after sutureless vitrectomy is usually transient, resolving within the first week of surgery as the sclerotomies heal sufficiently (Bamonte et al., 2011).

Bamonte et al. reported on the incidence of postoperative hypotony, defined as IOP of 5 mmHg or less, in their series of 25-gauge sutureless vitrectomy. They found that lens status, choice of tamponade, use of intravitreal triamcinolone, and reoperations to be independent risk factors for postoperative hypotony. Lens status has been shown to be a risk factor for postoperative hypotony with small gauge vitrectomy (Bamonte et al., 2011). Phakic eyes that did not undergo combined cataract extraction had a lower incidence of postoperative hypotony. This might be explained by the limited peripheral vitrectomy that is performed in these eyes to avoid lens contact.

Eyes undergoing primary small gauge vitrectomy have been shown to have a lower rate of postoperative hypotony compared to eye with previous vitrectomy (Bamonte et al., 2011; Shimada et al., 2006). It has been suggested that this finding could be a result of alterations in the elasticity and regenerative capacity of scleral tissue, leaving wounds in this tissue more prone to leakage. Additionally, revitrectomized eyes have more thorough vitreous removal, resulting in less vitreous plugging of the scleral wound. Vitreous base dissection has been shown to increase the rate of postoperative hypotony in 23-gauge surgery (Woo, et al., 2009).

Air or gas filled eyes have been shown to reduce the risk of hypotony (Bamonte et al., 2007; Shimada et al., 2006). It is felt that increased surface tension of air compared to BSS results in less leakage at the sclerotomy sites. This has led some surgeons to advocate a partial air-fluid exchange in eyes that undergo sutureless surgery, and that do not have a gas tamponade. The benefits of this technique on reducing the rate of postoperative hypotony has been demonstrated for both 25- and 23-gauge vitrectomy (Parolini et al,. 2010; Shimada et al. 2006).

7.2.2 Endophthalmitis

The rate of endophthalmitis with small gauge sutureless vitrectomy has been a concern. A very large retrospective study found a 12-fold increased risk of 25-gauge vitrectomy compared to 20-gauge vitrectomy (Kunimoto & Kaiser, 2007). In this study, Kunimoto and Kaiser reported an incidence of 0.23% (7/3,103 eyes) for 25-gauge and 0.018% (1/5,498 eyes) for 20-gauge vitrectomy. Limitations in the study included the retrospective nature and the use of triamcinolone in some cases of apparent endophthalmitis. Two other large studies have demonstrated a higher incidence with small gauge vitrectomy, but the differences were not significant (Scott et al., 2011; Chen, J. et al., 2009). Shimada et al., modified several aspects of 25-gauge vitrectomy, including creating shelved incisions, and found no difference in endophthalmitis rate compared to 20-gauge vitrectomy (Shimada et al., 2008).

The proposed mechanism for a possible higher risk of endophthalmitis is migration of bacteria from the ocular surface through the conjunctival and scleral wounds. Passage of India ink dye from the ocular surface into the scleral incision was demonstrated in rabbit eyes after 25- and 23-gauge incisions (Singh, 2008). The possible protective effect of angled incisions was demonstrated in this histopathologic study, and supported with clinical reports that had no endophthalmitis with shelved 25- and 23-gauge incisions (Gupta et al., 2008; Ibarra, 2005). It is possible that risks can be reduced with better wound construction using shelved incisions, conjunctival displacement, and prophylactic antibiotics.

7.2.3 Retinal detachment

It was hoped that the introduction of cannulas would reduce the incidence of retinal detachment due to less traction on the vitreous base during entry and removal of instruments. No large prospective trial has been performed to study this complication, but a very large retrospective study of 2,432 vitrectomies found no significant difference in the rates of retinal detachment between small gauge vitrectomy (23- and 25-gauge) and 20-gauge vitrectomy, or between 23- and 25-gauge vitrectomy (Rizzo et al., 2010). Reported rates of postoperative retinal detachment following 25-gauge vitrectomy have been similar to those reported for 20-gauge vitrectomy (Byeon, 2006; Ibarra, 2005). Table 3 summarizes the complications associated with small gauge vitrecomy.

Intraoperative	Postoperative
Hypotony	Hypotony
Intraocular Dislocation of Cannula	Endophthalmitis
Intrument Breakage	Retinal Detachment

Table 3. Complications of small gauge vitrectomy

8. Conclusion

Small gauge vitrectomy offers a number of advantages compared to the standard 20-gauge vitrectomy. Improvements in vitrector design and fluidics, as well as the development of a wide array of small gauge instruments, lasers, and illumination devices has significantly broadened the scope for small gauge vitrectomy surgery. As continued developments are made, 20-gauge vitrectomy may play a decreasing role in vitreoretinal surgery.

9. References

Abi-Ayed, N., Grange, J., Salle, M., & Kodjikian, L. (May 2011). Transretinal uveal melanoma biopsy with 25-gauge vitrectomy system. *Acta Ophthalmology,* 1755-3768 [E pub ahead of print]

Augustin, AJ. (2009) Historical overview of microincision surgery, In: *Vitreoretinal surgery progress III,* Rizzo S., Patelli, F. & Chow, DR, pp. (1-8) Springer, 1612-3212, Heidelberg, Germany

Brazitikos, PD. (2000). The expanding role of primary pars plana vitrectomy in the treatment of rhegamatogenous noncomplicated retinal detachment. *Semin Ophthalmol,* Vol. 15, No. 2, (June 2000), pp. (65-77), 0882-0538

Bamonte, G., Mura, M., & Tan, S. (2011). Hypotony after 25-gauge vitrectomy. *Am J* Ophthalmol, Vol. 151, (January 2011), pp. (156-160), 0002-9394

Byeon, SH, Chu, YK, Lee, SC, Koh, HJ, Kim, SS, & Kwon, OW. (2006). Problems associated with the 25-guage transconjunctival vitrectomy system during and after surgery. *Ophthalmologica*, Vol. 220, No. 4, (2006), pp. (259-265), 0030-3755

Charles, S., Calzada, J., Wood, B. (2007). *Vitreous Microsurgery* (Fourth edition), Lippincott Williams & Wilkins, 0-7817-6443-2, Philadelphia, PA.

Chen, CJ., Satofuka, S., Inoue, M., Ishida, S., Shinoda, K., & Tsubota, K. (2008). Suprachoroidal hemorrhage caused by breakage of a 25-gauge cannula. *Ophthalmic Surg Lasers Imaging*, Vol. 39, No. 4, (July 2008), pp. (323-324), 1542-8877

Chen, D., Lian, Y., Cui, L., Lu, F., Ke, Z., & Song, Z. Sutureless vitrectomy incision architecture in the immediate postoperative period evaluated in vivo using optical coherence tomography. *Ophthalmology*, Vol. 117, No. 10, (Oct 2010), pp. (2003-2009), 0161-6420

Chen, E. (2007). 25-gauge transconjunctival sutureless vitrectomy. *Curr Opin Ophthalmol*, Vol. 18, No. 3, (May 2007), pp (188-193), 1040-8738

Chen, JK, Khurana, RN, Nguyen, QD, & Do, DV. (2009). The incidence of endophthalmitis following transconjunctival sutureless 25- vs 20-gauge vitrectomy. *Eye (Lond)*, Vol. 23, No. 4, (Apr 2009), pp. (780-784), 0950-222X

Dalma-Weiszhausz, J., Gordon-Angelozzi, M., Ustariz-Gonzalez, O., & Suarez-Licona, A. (2008). Intraocular pressure rise during 25-gauge vitrectomy trocar placement. *Graefes Arch Clin Exp Ophthalmol*, Vol. 246, No. 2, (2008), pp. (187-189), 0721-832X

De Juan E. Jr & Hickingbotham, D. (1990) Refinements in microinstrumentation for vitreous surgery. *Am J Ophthalmol*, Vol.109, No. 2, (Feb 1990), pp. (218-20), 0002-9394

Eckardt, CM. (2005) Transconjunctival sutureless 23-gauge vitrectomy. *Retina*, Vol. 25, No. 2, (February/March 2005), pp.(208-11) 0275-004X

Elrich, R. & Polkinghorn, P. (2011) Small gauge vitrectomy in traumatic retinal detachment. *Clinical and experimental ophthalmology*, Vol. 39, No. 5, (July 2011), pp.(429-433), 1442-6404

Erakgun T., & Egrilmez S. (2009) Surgical outcomes of transconjunctival sutureless 23-gauge vitrectomy with silicone oil injection. *Indian J Ophthalmol*, Vol. 57, No. 2, (March-April 2009), pp. (105-109), 0301-4738

Fabian, ID & Moisseiev J. (2011) Sutureless vitrectomy: evolution and current practices. *British Journal of Ophthalmology*, Vol. 95, No. 3, (March 2011), pp.(318-324) 0007-1161

Fujii GY, de Juan E. Jr, Humayun MS, Pieramici, DJ, Chang, TS, Awh, C., Ng, E., Barnes, A., Wu, SL, & Sommerville, DN. (2002) A new 25-gauge instrument system for transconjunctival sutureless vitrectomy surgery. *Ophthalmology*, Vol. 109, No. 10, (October 2002), pp. (1807-12), 0161-6420

Gonzales, CR, Boshra J. & Schwartz, SD. (2006) 25-Gauge pars plicata vitrectomy for for stage 4 and 5 retinopathy of prematurity. *Retina* Vol. 26 Suppl 7 (Sept 2006) pp. (S42-S46), 0275-004X

Gonzales, CR, Singh, S., & Schwartz, SD. (2009). 25-Gauge vitrectomy for peadiatric vitreoretinal conditions. *Br J Ophthalmol*, Vol. 93, No. 6, (June 2009), pp. (787-790), 0007-1161

Gupta, O., Ho, A., & Kaiser, P. (2008). Short-term outcomes of 23-gauge pars plana vitrectomy. *Am J Ophthalmol*, Vol. 146, (August 2008), pp. (193-197), 0002-9394

Gupta, OP, Maguire, JI, Eagle, RC, Garg, SJ, & Gonye, GE. (2009). The competency of pars plana vitrectomy incisions: a comparative histologic and spectrophotometric analysis. *Am J Ophthalmol*, Vol. 147, No. 2, (Feb 2009), pp. (243-250), 0002-9394

Haas, A., Seidel, G., Steinbrugger, I., Maier, R., Gasser-Steiner, V., Wedrich, A., & Weger, M. (2010). Twenty-three-gauge and 20-gauge vitrectomy in epiretinal membrane surgery. *Retina*, Vol. 30, No. 1, (Jan 2010), pp. (112-116), 0275-004X

Hilton, G. (1985). A sutureless self-retaining infusion cannula for pars plana vitrectomy. *Am J Ophthalmol*, Vol. 99, No. 5, (May 1985), pp. (612), 0002-9394

Ho, LY, Walsh, MK & Hassan, TS. (2010) 25 Gauge pars plana vitrectomy for retained lens fragments. *Retina*, Vol. 30, No. 6, (June 2010), pp. (843- 849), 0275-004X

Hsu, J., Chen, E., Gupta, O., Fineman, M., Garg, S., & Regillo, C. (2008). Hypotony after 25-gauge vitrectomy using oblique versus direct cannula insertions in fluid-filled eyes. *Retina*, Vol. 28. No. 7, (July - August 2008), pp. (937-940), 0275-004X

Hubschman, JP, Gupta, A., Bouri,a DH, Culjat, M., Yu, F., & Schwartz, RD. (2008). 20-, 23-, 25-gauge vitreous cutters: performance and characteristics evaluation. *Retina*, Vol. 28, No. 2, (Feb 2008), pp.(249-257), 0275-004X

Ibarra, MS, Hermel, M., Prenner, JL, & Hassan, TS. (2005). Longer-term outcomes of transconjunctival sutureless 25-gauge vitrectomy. *Am J Opthalmol*, Vol. 139, No. 5, (May 2005), pp. (831-836), 0002-9394

Inoue, M., Noda, K., Ishida, S., Nagai, N., Imamura, Y., & Oguchi, Y. (2004) Intraoperative breakage of a 25-gauge vitreous cutter. *Am J Ophthalmol*, Vol. 138, No. 5, (Nov 2004), pp. (867-869), 0002-9394

Inoue, M., Shinoda, K., Shinoda, H., Kawamura, R., Suzuki, K., & Ishida, S. (2007). Two-step oblique incision during 25-gauge vitrectomy reduces incidence of postoperative hypotony. *Clin Experiment Ophthalmol*, Vol. 35, No. 8, (Nov 2007), pp (693-696), 1442-6404

Jackson, T. (2000). Modified sutureless sclerotomies in pars plana vitrectomy. *Am J Ophthalmol*, Vol. 129, No. 1, (Jan 2000), pp. (116-117), 0002-9394

Kadonosono, K., Yamakawa, T., Uchio, E., Yanagi, Y., Tamaki, Y., & Araie, M. (2006). Comparison of visual function after epiretinal membrane removal by 20-gauge and 25-gauge vitrectomy. *Am J Ophthalmol*, Vol. 142, (Septemper 2006), pp. (513-515), 0002-9394

Kasner, D. (1969). Vitrectomy: a new approach to management of vitreous. *Highlights Ophthalmol*, Vol. 11, (1969), pp. (304)

Kiss, S & Vavvas, D. (2008) 25 Gauge sutureless pars plana vitrectomy for removal of retained lens fragments and intraocular foreign bodies. *Retina*, Vol. 28, No.9, (October 2008), pp. (1346-1351), 0275-004X

Kongsap, P. (2010). Combined 20-gauge and 23-gauge pars plana vitrectomy for the management of posteriorly dislocated lens: a case series. *Clin Ophthalmol*, Vol. 4, (July 2010), pp. (625-628), 1177-5467

Kunikata, H., Uematsu, M., Nakazawa, T., & Fuse, N. (Feb 2011) Successful removal of large intraocular foreign body by 25 gauge microincision vitrectomy surgery. *Journal of Ophthalmology*, 2090-004X [E pub ahead of print]

Kunimoto, D. & Kaiser R. (2007). Incidence of endophthalmitis after 20- and 25-gauge vitrectomy. *Ophthalmol*, Vol. 114, (Dec 2007), pp. (2133-2137), 0161-6420

Leung, L., Nam, W., & Chang, S. (2010) Minimally invasive vitreoretinal surgery, In: *Minimally Invasive Ophthalmic Surgery*, Fine, IH & Mojon, DS, pp (217-225) Springer, 978-3-642-02601-0, Heidelberg, Germany

Lopez-Guajardo, L., Pareja-Esteban, J., & Teus-Guezala, MA. (2006). Oblique sclerotomy technique for prevention of incompetent wound closure in transconjunctival 25-gauge vitrectomy. *Am J Ophthalmol*, Vol. 141, (June 2006), pp. (1154-1156), 0002-9394

Machemer, R. (1995) The development of pars plana vitrectomy: a personal account. *Graefes Arch Clin Exp Ophthalmol.*, Vol. 233, No. 8, (Aug 1995), pp.(453-68), 0721-832X

Machemer R., & Hickingbotham D. (1985). The three-port microcannular system for closed vitrectomy. *Am J Ophthalmol*, Vol. 100, (October 1985), pp. (590-592), 0002-9394

Mangalhaes, O., Chong, L., DeBoer, C., Bhadri, P., Kerns, R., Barnes, A., Fang, S., Schor, P., & Humayun, M. (2009). Guillotine performance: duty cycle analysis of vitrectomy systems. *Retianl Cases & Brief Reports*, Vol. 3, No. 1, (Winter 2009), pp. (64-67), 1935-1089

Magalhaes, O Jr., Maia, M., Rodrigues, EB, Machado, L., Costa, EF, Maia, A., Moares-Filho, MN, Dib, E., & Farah, ME. (2011) Perspective on fluid and solid dynamics in different pars plana vitrectomy systems. *American Journal of Ophthalmology*, Vol. 151 No.3 , (March 2011) pp. (401-405e.1), 0002-9394

Mittra, RS & Pollak, JS. (2007). Preference and Trends Survey. Poster presented at: 25th Annual American Society of Retina Specialists Meeting, December 1-5, 2007; Indian Wells, CA). http://www.asrs.org; access for members only.

Misra, A., Ho-Yen, G., & Burton, RL. (2009). 23-gauge sutureless vitrectomy and 20-gauge vitrectomy: A case series comparison. *Eye*, Vol. 23, No. 5, (May 2009), pp. (1187-1191), 0950-222X

O'Malley C., & Heintz R. (1975). Vitrectomy with an alternative instrument system. *Ann Ophthalol*, Vol. 7, (April 1975), pp. (585-594), 0003-4886

Oshima, Y., Wakabayashi T., Sato, T, Ohji, M., & Tano, Y. (2010) A 27-gauge instrument system for transconjunctival sutureless microincision vitrectomy surgery. *Ophthalmology*, Vol. 117, No. 1 (January 2010), pp. (93-e102.e2), 0161-6420

Peyman, GA. (1990) A miniaturized vitrectomy system for vitreous and *retinal* biopsy. *Can J Ophthalmol*, Vol. 25, No. 6, (Oct 1990), pp. (285-6), 0008-4182

Recchia, F., Reichstein DA, & Kammer, JA. (2010). Small gauge vitrectomy in combination with glaucoma implant procedures. *Retina*, Vol. 30, No. 7, (July- August 2010), pp. (1152-54), 0275-004X

Recchia, FM, Scott, IU, Brown, GC, Brown, MM, Ho, AC, & Ip, MS. (2010) Small gauge pars plana vitrectomy. A report by the American Acadamy of Ophthalmology. *Ophthalmology*, Vol. 117, No. 9, (September 2010) pp. (1851-57), 0161-6420

Rizzo, S., Genovesi-Ebert, F., Murri, F., Belting, C., Vento, A., Cresti, F., & Manca, ML. (2006) 25-gauge sutureless vitrectomy and standard 20-gauge pars plana vitrectomy in idiopathic epiretinal membrane surgery: a comparative pilot study. *Graefes Arch Clin Exp Ophthalmol*, Vol. 244, (April 2006), pp. (472-479), 0721-832X

Rizzo, S., Patelli, F., Chow, DR. (2009). Essentials in Ophthalmology: *Vitreo-Retinal Surgery, Progress III*. Springer, ISBN 978-3-540-69461-8, Verlag, Berlin, Heidelberg, Germany

Rizzo, S., Beltling, C., Genovesi-Ebert, F., & Bartolo, E. (2010). Incidence of retinal detachment after small-incision, sutureless pars plana vitrectomy compared with conventional 20-gauge vitrectomy in macular hole and epiretinal membrane surgery. *Retina*, Vol. 20, No. 7, (July- August 2010), pp. (1065-1071), 0275-004X

Rodrigues EB, Meyer, CH, Mennel, S., & Farah, ME. (2007). Mechanisms of intravitreal toxicity of indocyanine green dye: implications for chemovitrectomy. *Retina*, Vol. 27, No. 7, (Sep 2007), pp. (958-970), 0275-004X

Rossi, T., Boccassini, B., Iossa, M., Lesnoni, G., & Tamburrelli, C. (2010) Choroidal hemorrhage drainage through 23 gauge vitrectomy cannulas. *Retina,* Vol. 30 No. 1, (January 2010), pp(174-176), 0275-004X

Schweitzer, C., Delyfer MN, Colin, J., & Korobelnik, JF. (2009) 23 gauge transconjunctival sutureless pars plana vitrectomy: results of a prospective study. *Eye,* Vol. 23, No. 12, (December 2009), pp. (2206-2214), 0950-222X

Scott, IU, Flynn, HW, Acar, N., Dev, S., Shaikh, S., Mittra RA, Arevalo, JF, Kychenthal, A., & Kunselman, A. (2011). Incidence of endophthalmitis after 20-gauge vs 23-gauge vs 25-gauge pars plana vitrectomy. *Graefes Arch Clin Exp Ophthalmol*, Vol. 249, No. 3, (Mar 2011), pp. (377-380), 0721-832X

Shimada, H., Nakashizuka, H., Mori, R., Mizutani, Y., & Hattori, T. (2006). 25-gauge scleral tunnel transconjunctival vitrectomy. *Am J Ophthalmol*, Vol. 142, (November 2006), pp. (871-873), 0002-9394

Shimada, H., Nakashizuka, H, Hattori, T., Mori, R., Mizutani, Y., & Yuzawa, M. (2008). Incidence of endophthalmitis after 20- and 25-gauge vitrectomy. *Ophthalmol*, Vol. 115, (December 2008), pp. (2215-2220), 0161-6420

Singh, A., Chen, JA, & Stewart, JM. (2008). Ocular surface fluid contamination of sutureless 25-gauge vitrectomy incisions. *Retina*, Vol. 28, No. 4, (April 2008), pp. (553-557), 0275-004X

Singh, RP, Bando, H., Brasil, OF, Williams, DR, & Kaiser, PK. (2008). Evaluation of wound closure using different incision techniques with 23-gauge and 25-gauge microincision vitrectomy systems. *Retina*, Vol. 28, No. 2, (Feb 2008), pp. (242-248), 0275-004X

Taban, M., Sharma, S., Ventura, A., & Kaiser, PK. (2009). Evaluation of wound closure in oblique 23-gauge sutureless sclerotomies with visante optical coherence tomography. *Am J Ophthalmol*, Vol. 147, No. 1, (Jan 2009), pp (101-107), 0002-9394

Thompson, JT. (2011) Advantages and limitations of small gauge vitrectomy. *Survey of ophthalmology,* Vol. 56, No. 2, (March- April), pp. (162-71), 0039-6257

Trikha, R., Yeung, CC, Modjtahedi, SP & Telander, DG. (2010) Evaluation of 25 gauge and 20 gauge vitrectomy on cell viability and diagnostic yield for B-cell lymphoma in culture using flow cytometry. *Retina,* Vol. 30, No. 9, (Oct 2010), pp. (1505-1510), 0275-004X

Warrier, SK, Jain, R., Gilhotra, JS, Newland, HS. (2008). Sutureless Vitrectomy. *Indian J Ophthalmol*, Vol 56, (November- December 2008), pp. (453-458), 0301-4738

Williams, GA. (2008) 25-, 23-, or 20-gauge instrumentation for vitreous surgery. *Eye,* Vol. 22, No. 10, (October 2010), pp. (1263-1266), 0950-222X

Williams, GA & Drenser, K. (2009) Epiretinal membrane surgery, In: *Surgical techniques in ophthalmology retina and vitreous surgery,* Bhavsar, AR, pp. (65-70) Saunders 978-1-4160-4206-8

Wong, RW, Kokame, GT, Mahmoud, TH, Mieler, WF, Tornambe, PE & McDonald, HR. (2010). Complications associated with clear corneal cataract wounds during vitrectomy. *Retina*, Vol. 30, No. 6, (June 2010), pp. 850-855, 0275-004X

Woo, SJ, Park, KH, Hwang, JM, Kim, JH, Yu, YS, & Chung, H. (2009). Risk factors associated with sclerotomy leakage and postoperative hypotony after 23-gauge transconjunctival sutureless vitrectomy. *Retina*, Vol. 29, No. 4, (Apr 2009), pp. (456-463), 0275-004X

Wu P., Tiong, IS, Chuang, YC, & Kuo, HK (2011). Twisting maneuver for sutureless vitrectomy trocar insertion to reduce intraoperative intraocular pressure rise. *Retina*, Vol. 31, No. 5, (May 2011), pp. (887-892), 0275-004X

Yeh, S., Weichel, E,. Faia, LJ, Albini, TA, Wroblewski, KK, Stetler-Stevenson, M., Ruiz, P, Sen, HN, Chan, CC, & Nussenblat, RB . (2010) 25- gauge transconjunctival sutureless vitrectomy for the diagnosis of intraocular lymphoma. *British Journal of Ophthalmology*, Vol. 94, No. 5, (May 2010), pp. (633-638) 0007-1161

5

Postoperative Tamponade and Positioning Restrictions After Macular Hole Surgery

Yuhei Hasegawa, Yasutaka Mochizuki and Yasuaki Hata
Department of Ophthalmology,
Graduate School of Medical Sciences, Kyushu University
Japan

1. Introduction

Idiopathic macular hole is a defect of the foveal retina involving its full thickness from the internal limiting membrane to the outer segment of the photoreceptor layer. According to the Gass Classification System, macular holes can be classified into four stages as shown in Table 1 (Gass, 1995).

Stage 1a	Foveal detachment. Macular cyst. Tangential vitreous traction results in the elevation of the fovea.
Stage 1b	As the foveal retina elevates to the level of the perifoveal, the yellow dot of xanthophyll pigment changes to a donut shaped yellow ring.
Stage 2	A full-thickness macular hole less than 400 μm in size.
Stage 3	A full-thickness macular hole which is greater than 400 μm in size and is still with partial vitreomacular adhesion/traction.
Stage 4	A full-thickness macular hole exists in the presence of a complete separation of the vitreous from the macula and the optic disc.

Table 1. Gass classification of idiopathic macular hole

Indications of the surgical management of macular hole are based on the presence of a full-thickness defect (stage 2 or higher). Once this defect has developed, the potential for spontaneous resolution is low. Since the initial report by Kelly NE, the surgical technique of idiopathic macular hole has been improved (Kelly & Wendel, 1991). Currently, the most standard surgical technique for the treatment of idiopathic macular hole is pars plana vitrectomy with peeling of the internal limiting membrane and intraocular gas tamponade followed by prone positioning (Schaal et al., 2006). However, the mechanisms of macular hole closure have not been fully elucidated.There are two theories accounting for the process of macular hole closure and the role of the tamponade material. One is the buoyancy theory and the other is the isolation theory (Gupta, 2009). The buoyancy theory is based on the idea that the buoyancy force 'presses' the edges of the macular hole. Thus, prone positioning is considered necessary for closure of the macular hole. On the other hand, the isolation theory, which is also called 'waterproofing', is based on the idea that the tamponade material 'plug' the macular hole and subretinal fluid is absorbed by retinal pigment epithelium (Goldbaum et al., 1998). macular hole might thus be closed without prone positioning as long as there is adequate isolation of aqueous humor (Figure 1).

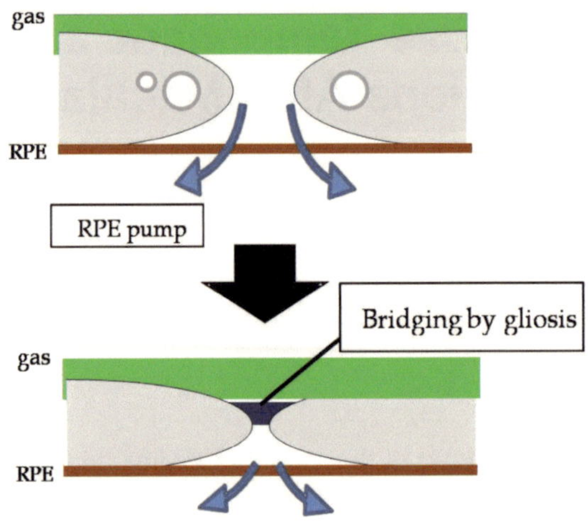

Fig. 1. Scheme of the isolation theory. RPE; retinal pigment epithelium

It has been reported that the prognostic factors of macular hole surgery were the stage of macular hole and hole diameter, but it remains unclear which is the most important factor for surgical outcome of macular hole (Ellis et al., 2000; Ullrich et al., 2002; Wells & Gregor, 1996). In our previous study, hole diameter was the most important prognostic factor among them (Hasegawa et al., 2009). And, the high closure rates were recently achieved regardless of tamponade material, so, there are many reports regarding the selection of tamponade material and the necessity of positioning restrictions after macular hole surgery. The tamponade materials have several features, and the extent of positioning restrictions vary among them. In this review, we will discuss recent advances in tamponade materials and positioning restrictions after macular hole surgery.

2. Tamponade materials after vitrectomy for macular hole

Sulfur hexafluoride (SF_6), octafluoropropane (C_3F_8), hexafluoroethane (C_2F_6), room air and silicone oil are common tamponade materials (Goldbaum et al., 1998; Park et al., 1999; Thompson et al., 1996; Tornambe et al., 1997). Although the exact mechanism of the tamponade material is controversial, it is thought that the longer the tamponade material stays in the operated eye, the surer the effect of tamponade, but, confirmation of macular hole closure and visual rehabilitation is delayed while tamponade material is covering the macular region. In addition, the residual tamponade material in the vitreous cavity impedes return to normal activity, especially in the case of long-acting gas or silicone oil. For example, patients with a gas bubble in their eyes cannot generally undertake air travel, and a refractive hyperopic shift occurs in the eyes filled with silicone oil. Additionally when using silicone oil, patients need to undergo re-operation for later removal. Frequently it takes over one week before one is able to examine the state of the macular regions through aqueous humor when using long-acting gas. Using room air, this generally becomes possible in about 3 days. There are also various opinions regarding the necessity of positioning restrictions after macular hole surgery. Positions include prone (face-down), seated, lateral and avoid spine (not to lie flat on the back) positioning (Chignell & Billingto, 1986; Krohn, 2005; Madula & Costen, 2008; Merkur & Tuli, 2007; Minihan t al., 1997; Thompson et al., 1994; Tornambe et al., 1997; Tranos et al., 2007). It has been thought that macular hole is expected to close when adequately isolated from aqueous humor (the isolation theory) (Goldbaum et al., 1998). Probably, the surest positioning for isolation of macular hole is prone positioning. However, it is better to shorten the prone positioning period as much as possible because most patients suffer from discomfort and noncompliance when continuing the such positioning for extended periods. Nevertheless, it is important to maintain adequate closure rates. There are many reports describing how long a duration of prone positioning is required (Krohn, 2005; Sato & Isomae, 2003; Takahashi & Kishi, 2000; Thompson et al., 1996; Isomae et al., 2002). Opinions range from 1day to 4 weeks. In addition, there are several reports of successful macular hole closure without prone positioning (Merkur & Tuli, 2007; Tornambe et al., 1997; Tranos et al., 2007). The selection of tamponade material has relevance to the type of positioning restrictions. That is to say, the positioning restriction could be eased when using a gas with extended duration in the operated eye. The choice of tamponade material or positioning after macular hole surgery is dependent upon many issues, such as the opinion of surgeons or the condition of patients. Which is the best tamponade material after vitrectomy for macular hole? Which positioning is the most adequate for both the treatment of macular hole and the benefit of patients? In the present issue, we will review the various points of view.

3. Usefulness of room air as a tamponade material

It was reported that a long-acting intraocular gas tamponade is a substantially higher success rate for macular hole surgery as compared with a short-acting one (Thompson et al., 1994). However, gas tamponade may cause several side effects including intraocular pressure elevation and retinal artery occlusion due to its expansion when not diluted appropriately. Although it is generally known that SF_6 should be diluted to 20 %, and that C_3F_8 to 12 %, intraocular pressure elevation actually occurred sometimes. And postoperative cataract development is also worried for phakic eyes, especially for traumatic macular holes of young patients who should not undergo cataract surgery simultaneously. On the other hand, complications were rare according to our experiences when air was used as a tmaponade material because it is not expanded and is absorbed faster than long-acting gas. Indeed, the usefulness of air as a tamponade material after vitrectomy for macular hole has been recently reported (Hasegawa et al., 2009; Krohn , 2005; Sato et al., 2003). Hikichi et al. reported that macular holes closed successfully after the primary vitrectomy in all eyes using air tamponade (Hikichi et al., 2011). Their studies reported high closure rates of 91 % to 100 %. We also investigated the tamponade effect of air and the shortening of the prone positioning period (Hasegawa et al., 2009). In this study, the macular hole closure was postoperatively confirmed by optical coherence tomography once the macular area could be precisely examined through aqueous humor. At that time, prone positioning was terminated. The primary closure rate was 92.3 % after 3.83 days of prone positioning and is consistent with other tamponade materials. Thus, air may have equivalent tamponade effect after macular hole surgery compared with other tamponade materials (Da Mata et al., 2004; Haritoglou et al., 2006; Lai & Williams, 2007). Moreover, air with its short duration in the postoperative eye can result in more rapid visual rehabilitation and earlier detailed evaluation of the macular region. According to the isolation theory, the buoyancy force may not be as important for macular hole closure, and macular hole is likely to close when isolated adequately from aqueous humor (Stopa et al., 2007). However, we request patients to maintain prone positioning for at least several hours after their operation. At this time, there is insufficient evidence to allow firm conclusions as to whether prone positioning after macular hole surgery influences closure rates. More recently, the early postoperative state of macular hole can be investigated because imaging of the macular region through gas bubble may now be obtained by advances in optical coherence tomography technology (Eckardt et al., 2008; Kasuga et al., 2000; Masuyama et al., 2009).

4. Trial to shorten prone positioning period

It is thought that prone positioning is not inherently necessary (Gupta, 2009). Many macular holes, especially small size holes, are expected to close without prone positioning according to the isolation theory. Although we think that prone positioning is the best way for optimizing isolation of macular hole, we also think that the prone positioning period should be shortened as much as possible. So, we performed a trial to shorten the prone positioning period while maintaining sufficient closure rates. Our method is to terminate the prone positioning once we can confirm anatomical closure of the hole using optical coherence tomography even under retained tamponade material. First, optical coherence tomography images were obtained 6 hours after vitrectomy. When we could not confirm that the hole was closed, optical coherence tomography images were obtained again 24 hours after operation. And, we repeated this procedure every 24 hours till the hole closure was confirmed. We present the results in this chapter. This study was approved by the Institutional Review Board and performed in accordance with the ethical standards of the 1989 Declaration of Helsinki. Written informed consents were obtained from all patients enrolled in this study. This study consists of a prospective consecutive series of macular hole patients after vitrectomy with internal limiting membrane peeling. A total of 16 eyes (5 male eyes and 11 female eyes) of 16 patients and aged 55-83 years (average 66 years) were identified. Figure 2 is the representative image of postoperative macular region in air-filled eye.

We judged the macular hole to be closed when the edges of hole were connected in all slices of spectral-domain-optical coherence tomography, and prone positioning was terminated 6 hours after operation in this case. The optical coherence tomography image in 11 eyes (68.8 %) could be obtained at the day of vitrectomy and the prone positioning was terminated in 72.8 % of them (50 % of all cases) since the hole closure was confirmed by all slices. The hole was finally judged to be closed or not to be under the presence of air in 15 eyes/ 16 eyes (93.8 %) (Table 2).

Day from operation		Closed eyes (Closure rates)
Operation's day	11/16 eyes (68.8 %)	8 eyes (50 %)
One day	13/16 eyes (81.3 %)	13 eyes (81.3%)
Two days	15/16 eyes (93.8 %)	14 eyes (87.5%)

Table 2. Cases which their macular region could be confirmed by spectral-domain-optical coherence tomography under air bubble

As shown in Figure 3, prone positioning could be terminated in less than 24 hours in 13 eyes (81.3 %).

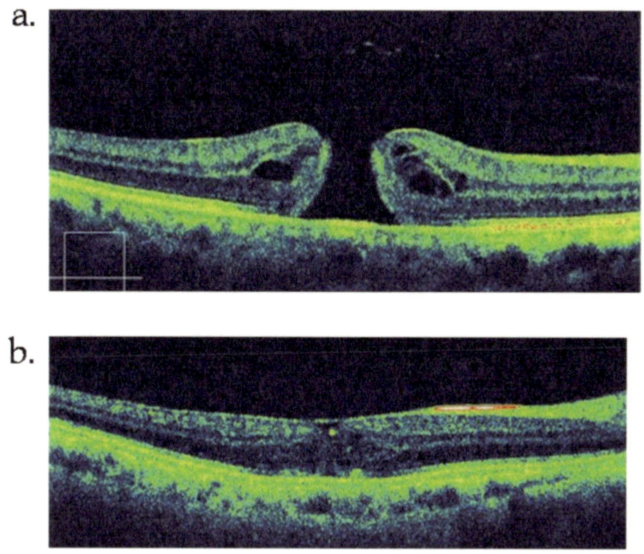

Fig. 2. Representative images of preoperative macular hole (a) and postoperative macular region in air-filled eye (b)

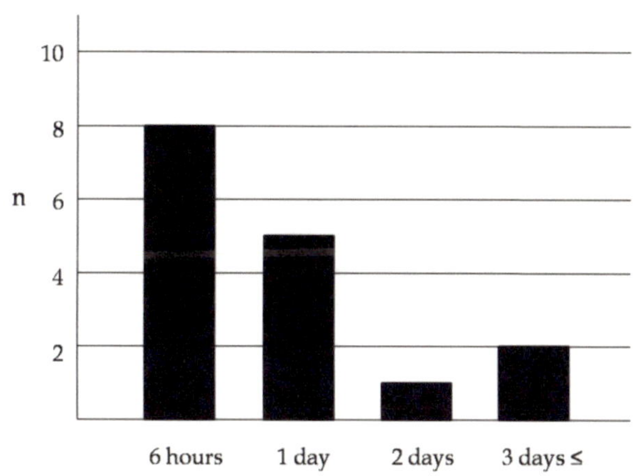

Fig. 3. Period of prone positioning

Compared with our previous report, the primary closure rate, which is 87.5 % (14 of 16 eyes), was almost equal and the mean prone positioning period, which is 2.24 days, in this study was shorter. (Hasegawa et al., 2009) One unclosed case was finally closed after the retinal stretch and the exchange of vitreous cavity by 20 % SF_6 at 5 days after operation with 1 day prone positioning after reoperation. In another unclosed case, although we once judged the hole to be closed by optical coherence tomography images and the prone positioning was terminated as shown in Figure 4, the patient restarted prone positioning next day because the hole was confirmed not to be closed.

It was finally closed without reoperation for 4 days prone positioning. Thus it appears easier to judge that macular hole is not closed than it is to determine if the macular hole is closed.

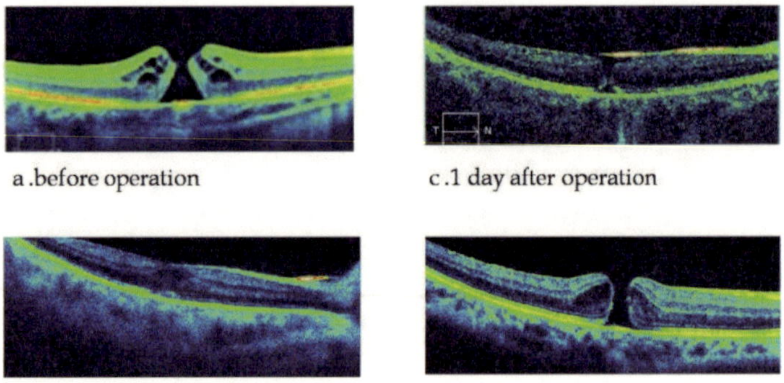

a .before operation

c .1 day after operation

b .6 hours after operation

d .2 days after operation

Fig. 4. A case in whom prone positioning was continued for 4 days

The thinly sliced optical coherence tomography images and re-examinations are necessary for surer confirmation of macular hole closure when using this method. The daily images of optical coherence tomography monitoring may become a help to resolve the healing procedure of macular hole. This study is limited by the few cases evaluated and further investigation is necessary.

5. Discussion

There has been no absolute generally accepted answer with regard to which is the best tamponade material after vitrectomy for macular hole. Widely used tamponade materials include SF_6, C_3F_8, C_2F_6, air and silicone oil. Silicone oil usually is not selected after macular hole surgery except in the case of macular hole with retinal detachment (Wolfensberger TJ & Gonvers M, 1999). After Tornambe et al. reported that they had achieved hole closure in 79% of their cases using a 15 % C_3F_8 without prone positioning, many studies have been performed concerning tamponade materials and posturing (Tornambe et al. 1997). So far, a long-acting gas has been used more frequently than air. However, usefulness of air was recently investigated. At first, Park et al. used air tamponade with 4 days prone positioning and observed hole closure in 91 % (Park et al., 1999). A closure rate over 90 % has been reported using air, including our previous report (Hasegawa et al., 2009; Hikichi et al., 2011; Sato et al., 2003). The recent views concerning management after macular hole surgery can be divided into two general approaches. One is using long-acting gas with loose positioning restrictions. The other is using air with prone positioning while shortening the period as much as possible. In our current treatment for macular hole, we use air tamponade with prone positioning and terminate the prone positioning once we can confirm anatomical closure using optical coherence tomography under the presence of air. The closure rate of 87.5 % was almost equal to the result of Eckardt et al. in which they used similar methods as ours (Eckardt et al., 2008). In previous studies, it has been reported that the prognostic factors of macular hole surgery were the stage of macular hole, hole diameter, age of the macular hole and axial length (Ellis et al., 2000; Suda et al., 2011; Ullrich et al., 2002; Wells & Gregor, 1996). There were two cases required prone positioning over 3 days in this study. One case was an old (5 years) and large hole (870 μm) and the other was also an old hole (15 years). In order to increase closure rates more, it might be better to use long-acting gas as tamponade material for keeping macular region dry for longer time and perform the additional treatment such as retinal stretch in cases which have bad prognostic factors, such as large diameter or long axial length (Wells & Gregor, 1996; Suda et al., 2011). We assume hole closure once there is connection of hole edges. However, there was one case where the hole was actually not closed even though we had judged it to be closed as shown in Figure 4. Arima et al. reported the supportive usefulness of fundus autofluorescence for confirming macular hole closure (Arima et al., 2009).

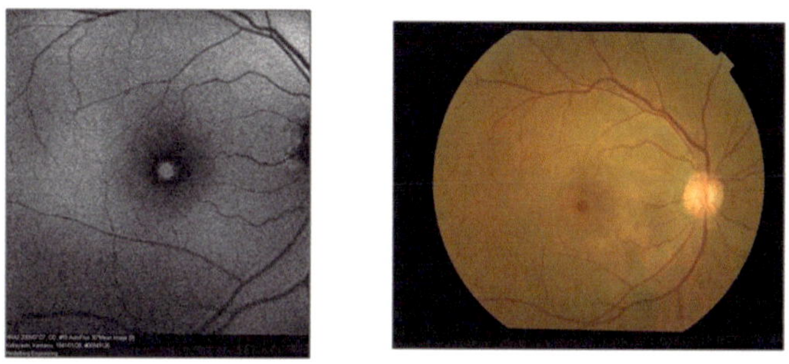

a. Representative FAF image

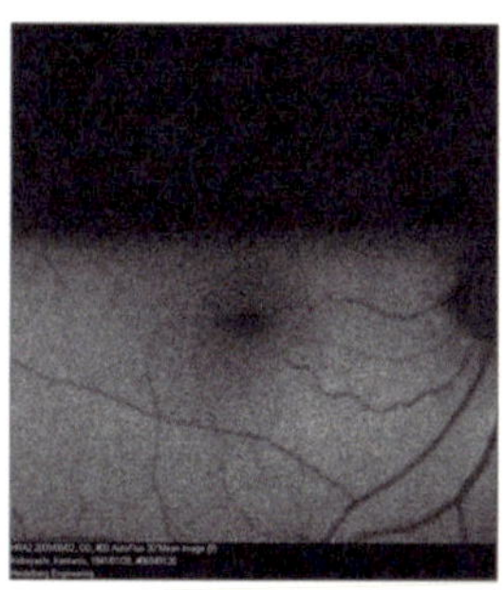

b. Postoperative FAF image of closed case

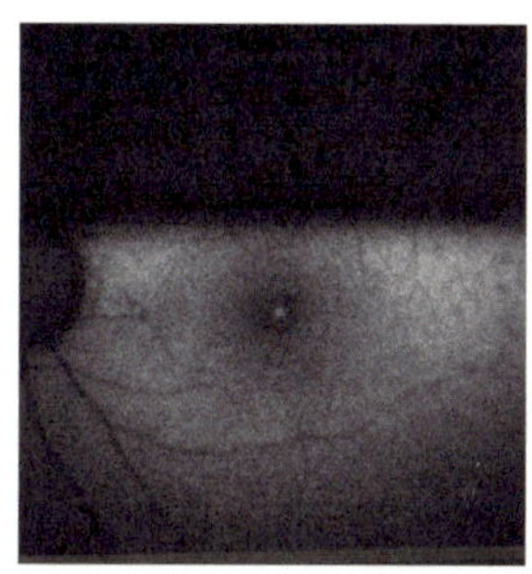

c. Postoperative FAF image of unclosed case

Fig. 5. Representative fundus autofluorescence(FAF) images

a. Representative preoperative FAF image and Fundus Photography
b. Postoperative FAF image of closed case
c. Postoperative FAF image of unclosed case

As shown in Figure 5, unclosed macular hole reveals a bright hyperfluorescence spot and a tiny space of retina which can be overlooked by optical coherence tomography can be detected by fundus autofluorescence imaging. However, early closure of macular hole cannot be confirmed using fundus autofluorescence imaging because it cannot be obtained through a gas/air bubble. There are several differences such as half-life, side effects and the way of positioning restriction, between long-acting gas and air and cases of macular hole can also vary substantially. For example, there are some instances in which patients cannot maintain prone positioning due to their general conditions. In addition, the methods of macular hole treatment have been increasing because small-gauge transconjunctival vitrectomy is gaining wide acceptance recently (Fujii et al., 2002; Fujii et al., 2002). It is important for each operator to select the tamponade material and posturing which is thought to be the most suitable for each patient. The role of tamponade material has been widely debated. Gupta mentioned the comparison of two theories, namely the buoyancy theory and the isolation theory, regarding the role of the tamponade material in his review manuscript (Gupta, 2009). The former is based on the idea that the buoyancy force (floating force) may be necessary to maintain a mechanical pressure against the hole edges. With regard to the buoyancy theory, it is by that buoyancy forces cannot be of significance in gas-filled eyes immediately after operation (Stopa et al., 2007). Indeed, many studies report equivalent macular hole closure rates using long-acting gas or silicone oil (which has very little buoyancy force) without prone posturing. This seems to support the isolation theory, but not the buoyancy theory. The latter is based on the idea that the gas bubble may provide a scaffold to support formation of a bridging preretinal membrane and that subretinal fluid will be eliminated via the retinal pigment epithelium pump when tamponade materials ensure the macula remains dry (Figure 1) (Berger & Brucker, 1998; Gupta, 2009). However, it is rather difficult to document the occurrence of the healing responses, such as a cellular migration (Charles, 2004). Recently, several reports have confirmed that holes can close as early as 1 day after surgery using optical coherence tomography images under the gas/air bubble (Jumper et al., 2000; Satchi & Patel, 2002). According to the isolation theory, prone posturing seems not to be necessary in early closed cases.

6. Conclusion

There are numerous opinions concerning the selection of tamponade material and the necessity of prone positioning after macular hole surgery. Different cases may need to be approached in different ways. It is important to select the tamponade material and posturing approach in relation to each individual situation. The confirmation of early macular hole closure using optical coherence tomography imaging under the gas/air bubble can be a great help in modifying subsequent care. Further investigations are required to maximize macular hole closure rates while shortening the period of postoperative position restrictions.

7. References

Arima, M.; Miyazaki, M.; Kohno, R.; Hata, Y. & Ishibashi, T. (2009) An early "reopening" case of idiopathic macular hole; supportive usefulness of fundus autofluorescence. *Graefes Arch Clin Exp Ophthalmol* Vol.247, No.5, pp. 711-714, ISSN 0721-832X

Berger, JW. & Brucker, AJ. (1998) The magnitude of the bubble buoyant pressure: implications for macular hole surgery. *Retina* Vol.18, No.1, pp. 86-88, ISSN 0275-004X

Charles S (2004) An engineering approach to vitreoretinal surgery. *Retina* Vol.24, No.3, pp. 435-444, ISSN 0275-004X

Chignell, AH. & Billington, B. (1986) The treatment of macular holes by pars plana vitrectomy and internal air/SF6 exchange. *Graefes Arch Clin Exp Ophthalmol* Vol.224, No.1, pp. 67-68, ISSN 0721-832X

Da Mata, AP.; Burk, SE.; Foste, RE.; Riemann, CD.; Petersen, MR.; Nehemy, MB. & Augsburger, JJ. (2004) Long-term follow-up of indocyanine green-assisted peeling of the retinal internal limiting membrane during vitrectomy surgery for idiopathic macular hole repair. *Ophthalmology* Vol.111, No.12, pp. 2246-2253

Eckardt, C.; Eckert, T.; Eckardt, U.; Porkert, U. & Gesser, C. (2008) Macular hole surgery with air tamponade and optical coherence tomography-based duration of face-down positioning. *Retina* Vol.28, No.8, pp. 1087-1096, ISSN 0275-004X

Ellis, JD.; Malik, TY.; Taubert, MA.; Barr, A. & Baines, PS. (2000) Surgery for full-thickness macular holes with short-duration prone posturing: results of a pilot study. *Eye* Vol.14, Jun, Pt 3A, pp. 307-312, ISSN 0950-222X

Fujii, GY.; De Juan, E. Jr.; Humayun, MS.; Chang, TS.; Pieramici, DJ.; Chang, TS.; Awh, C.; Ng, E.; Barnes, A.; Wu, SL. & Sommerville, DN. (2002) A new 25-gauge instrument system for transconjunctival sutureless vitrectomy surgery. *Ophthalmology* Vol.109, No.10, pp. 1807-1812

Fujii, GY.; De Juan, E. Jr.; Humayun, MS.; Chang, TS.; Pieramici, DJ.; Barnes, A. & Kent, D. (2002) Initial experience using the transconjunctival sutureless vitrectomy system for vitreoretinal surgery. *Ophthalmology* Vol.109, No.10, pp. 1814-1820

Gass, JD. (1995) Reappraisal of biomicroscopic classification of stages of development of a macular hole. *Am J Ophthalmol* Vol.119, No.6, pp. 752-759, ISSN 0002-9394

Goldbaum, MH.; McCuen, BW.; Hanneken, A.; Burgess, SK. & Chen, HH. (1998) Silicone oil tamponade to seal macular holes without position restrictions. *Ophthalmology* Vol.105, No.11, pp. 2140-2148

Gupta, D. (2009) Face-down posturing after macular hole surgery: a review. *Retina* Vol.29, No.4, pp. 430-443, ISSN 0275-004X

Haritoglou, C.; Reiniger, IW.; Schaumberger, M.; Gass, CA.; Priglinger, SG. & Kampik, A. (2006) Five-year follow-up of macular hole surgery with peeling of the internal limiting membrane: update of a prospective study. *Retina* Vol.26, No.6, pp. 618-622, ISSN 0275-004X

Hasegawa, Y.; Hata, Y.; Mochizuki, Y.; Arita, R.; Kawahara, S.; Kita, T.; Noda, Y, & Ishibashi, T. (2009) Equivalent tamponade by air compared with SF_6 after macular hole surgery. *Graefes Arch Clin Exp Ophthalmol* Vol.247, No.11, pp. 1455-1459, ISSN 0721-832X

Hikichi, T.; Kosaka, S.; Takami, K.; Ariga, H.; Ohtsuka, H.; Higuchi, M.; Matsushita, T. & Matsushita, R. (2011) 23- and 20-gauge vitrectomy with air tamponade with combined phacoemulsification for idiopathic macular hole: a single-surgeon study.vitreous surgery. *Am J Ophthalmol* Vol.152, No.1, pp. 114-121, ISSN 0002-9394

Isomae, T.; Sato, Y. & Shimada, H. (2002) Shortening the duration of prone positioning after macular hole surgery comparison between 1-week and 1-day prone positioning. *Jpn J Ophthalmol* Vol.46, No.1, pp. 84-88, ISSN 0021-5155

Jumper, JM.; Gallemore, RP.; McCuen, BW. 2nd. & Toth, CA. (2000) Features of macular hole closure in the early post-operative period using optical coherence tomography. *Retina* Vol.20, No.3, pp.232-237, ISSN 0275-004X

Kasuga, Y.; Arai, J.; Akimoto, M. & Yoshimura, N. (2000) Optical coherence tomograghy to confirm early closure of macular holes. *Am J Ophthalmol* Vol.130, No.5, pp. 675-676, ISSN 0002-9394

Kelly, NE. & Wendel, RT. (1991) Vitreous surgery for idiopathic macular holes. Results of a pilot study. *Arch Ophthalmol* Vol.109, No.5, pp. 654-659, ISSN 0003-9950

Krohn, J. (2005) Duration of face-down positioning after macular hole surgery: a comparison between 1 week and 3 days. *Acta ophthalmol Scand* Vol.83, No.3, pp. 289-292, ISSN 1395-3907

Lai, MM. & Williams, GA. (2007) Anatomical and visual outcomes of idiopathic macular hole surgery with internal limiting membrane removal using low-concentration indocyanine green. *Retina* Vol.27, No.4, pp. 477-482, ISSN 0275-004X

Madula, IM. & Costen, M. (2008) Functional outcome and patient preferences following combined phaco-vitrectomy for macular hole without prone posturing. *Eye* Vol.22, Jun, pp. 1050-1053, ISSN 0950-222X

Masuyama, K.; Yamakiri, K.; Arimura, N.; Sonoda, Y.; Doi, N. & Sakamoto, T. (2009) Posturing time after macular hole surgery modified by optical coherence tomography images: a pilot study. *Am J Ophthalmol* Vol.147, No.3, pp. 481-488, ISSN 0002-9394

Merkur, AB. & Tuli, R. (2007) Macular hole repair with limited nonsupine positioning. *Retina* Vol.27, No.3, pp. 365-369, ISSN 0275-004X

Minihan, M.; Goggin, M. & Cleary, PE. (1997) Surgical management of macular holes: results using gas tamponade alone, or in combination with autologous platelet concentrate, or transforming growth factor beta 2. *Br J Ophthalmol* Vol.81, No.12, pp. 1073-1079, ISSN 0007-1161

Park, DW.; Sipperley, JO.; Sneed, SR.; Dugel, PU. & Jacobsen, J. (1999) Macular hole surgery with internal-limiting membrane peeling and intravitreous air. *Ophthalmology* Vol.106, No.7, pp. 1392-1398

Satchi, K. & Patel, CK. (2002) Posterior chamber compartments demonstrated by optical coherence tomography, in silicone filled eyes, following macular hole surgery. *Clin Experiment Ophthalmol*. Vol.33, No.6, pp.619-622, ISSN 1442-6404

Sato, Y. & Isomae, T. (2003) Macular hole surgery with internal limiting membrane removal, air tamponade, and 1-day prone positioning. *Jpn J Ophthalmol* Vol.47, No.1, pp. 503-506, ISSN 0021-5155

Schaal, KB.; Bartz-schmidt, KU. & Dithmar, S. (2006) Current strategies for macular hole surgery in Germany, Australia and Switzerland. *Ophthalmologue* Vol.103, No.5, pp. 922-926, ISSN 1433-0423

Stopa, M.; Lincoff, A. & Lincoff, H. (2007) Analysis of forces acting upon submacular hemorrhage in pneumatic displacement. *Retina* Vol.27, No.3, pp. 370-374, ISSN 0275-004X

Suda, K.; Hangai, M. & Yoshimura, N. (2011) Axial length and outcomes of macular hole surgery assessed by spectral-domain optical coherence tomography. *Am J Ophthalmol* Vol.151, No.1, pp. 118-127, ISSN 0002-9394

Takahashi, H. & Kishi, S. (2000) Tomographic features of early macular hole closure after vitreous surgery. *Am J Ophthalmol* Vol.130, No.2, pp. 192-196, ISSN 0002-9394

Thompson, JT.; Glaser, BM.; Sjaarda, RN.; Murphy, RP. & Hanham, A. (1994) Effects of intraocular bubble duration in the treatment of macular holes by vitrectomy and transforming growth factor-beta 2. *Ophthalmology* Vol.101, No.7, pp. 1195-1200

Thompson, JT.; Smiddy, WE.; Glaser, BM.; Sjaarda, RN. & Flynn, HW. Jr. (1996) Intraocular tamponade duration and success of macular hole surgery. *Retina* Vol.16, No.5, pp. 373-382, ISSN 0275-004X

Tornambe, PE.; Poliner, LS. & Grote, K. (1997) Macular hole surgery without face-down positioning. A pilot study. *Retina* Vol.17, No.3, pp. 179-185, ISSN 0275-004X

Tranos, PG.; Peter, NM.; Nath, R.; Singh, M.; Dimitrakos, S.; Charteris, D. & Kon, C. (2007) Macular hole surgery without prone positioning. *Eye* Vol.21, No.6, pp. 802-806, ISSN 0950-222X

Ullrich, S.; Haritoglou, C.; Gass, C.; Schaumberger, M.; Ulbig, MW. & Kampik, A. (2002) Macular hole size as a prognostic factor in macular hole surgery. *Br J Ophthalmol* Vol.86, No.4, pp. 390-393, ISSN 0007-1161

Wells, JA. & Gregor, ZJ. (1996) Surgical treatment of full-thickness macular holes using autologous serum. *Eye* Vol.10, No.5, pp. 593-599, ISSN 0950-222X

Wolfensberger, TJ. & Gonvers, M. (1999) Long-term follow-up of retinal detachment due tomacular hole in myopic eyes treated by temporary silicone oil tamponade and laser photocoagulation. *Ophthalmology* Vol.106, No.9, pp. 1786-1791

6

Macular Edema Surgical Treatment

Jin Ma
Eye Center of Second Associated Hospital, Zhejiang University College of Medicine China

1. Introduction

Macular edema (ME) represents a common final pathway of many intraocular and systemic diseases, which characterized by the accumulation of extracellular fluid in Henle's layer and the inner nuclear layer of the retina. ME can cause severe visual disturbances and be considered to be multifactorial and difficult to treat. It may be most commonly seen following diabetic retinopathy, retinal vascular occlusion, intraocular surgery, uveitis, pigmentary degeneration, and/or vitreoretinal traction syndrome. The pathogenesis of ME involves the interplay of several affected factors, including the breakdown of the inner and outer blood retinal barriers, release of biochemical messengers, tissue hypoxia, retinal circulatory changes, and vitreous traction. Although medications and some other therapeutic methods are effective in some cases, they cannot be the best treatment due to adverse effects or lack of durability. Thus, the role of the vitreous in the development of ME has received attention. Abnormal glycation cross-linking of vitreal collagen has been found in the vitreous of ME cases. The abnormal collagen structure can destabilize the vitreous, leading to traction on the macula [1-7], which may distort the BRB and result in ME. On the other hand, the breakdown of the blood retinal barriers can lead to a high concentration of vasopermeable and chemoattractant factors in the posterior vitreous [8]. This pool of agents can cause cell migration to the posterior hyaloid. Contraction of these cells could lead to macular traction with possible development of a shallow macular detachment and exacerbation of ME [9,10]. (Fig. 1) Thus, we discuss the possibility of surgical treatment for ME in the following.

2. Vitrectomy

The role of the vitreous in the formation of DME has been recognized. A few study shows that in various disorders, including aphakia, uveitis, branched vein occlusion, and diabetic retinopathy, the vitreous could remain attached to the macula with the firm vitreomacular adhesions, which could cause traction on the inner limiting membrane (ILM) of the macula and exacerbate the ME. When the vitreous was either completely liquefied (Stickler syndrome and high myopia) or the hyaloid face had completely detached from the retina, the ME could be elimilated [11-12]. This finding demonstrated that the vitreous played a role in the development of ME and suggested that complete posterior vitreous detachment had a protective effect against the development of ME. Thus, the vitreous could play a role in exacerbating the ME, and the treatment of vitrectomy with separation of the posterior hyaloid from the macula could be beneficial.

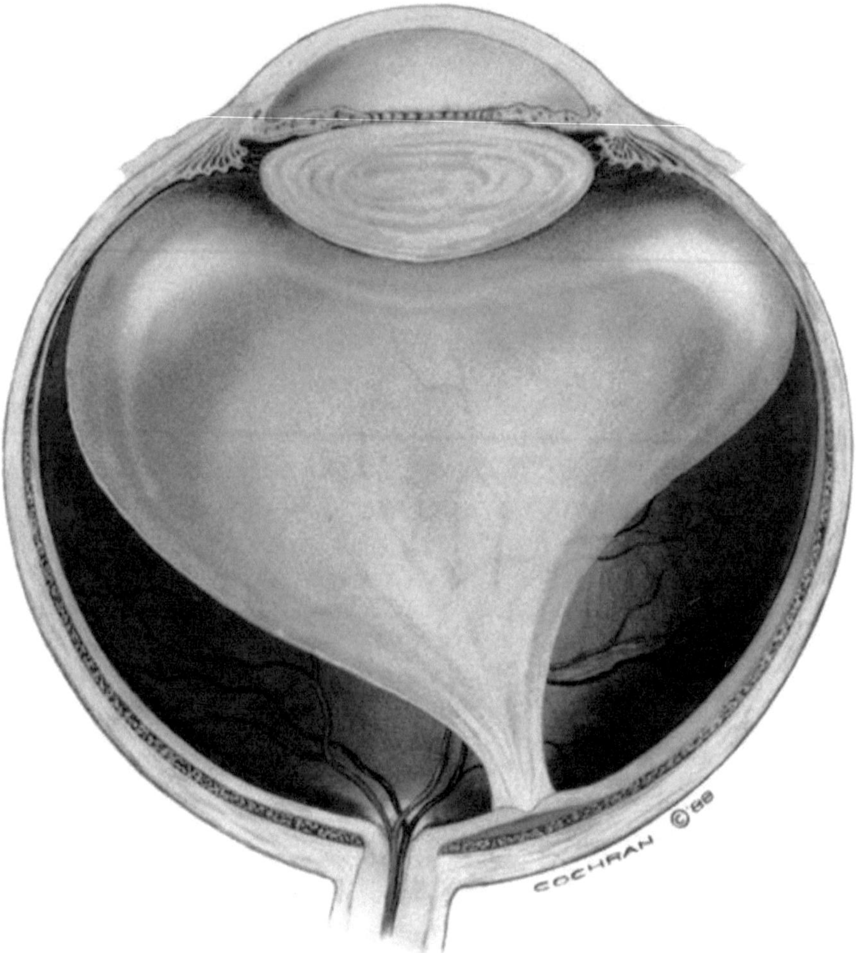

Fig. 1. Vitreomacular traction for macular edema. (From Margherio RR, Trese MT, Margherio AR et al: Surgical management of vitreomacular traction syndromes. Ophthalmology 1989;96:1439)

Why does vitrectomy and hyaloid removal could relieve ME? The release of vitreomacular traction is one obvious mechanism. The tractional force of the posterior hyaloid to the macula as seen in vitreomacular traction may be important in the pathogenesis of ME which has been well-demonstrated by optical coherence tomography [13]. In addition, vitrectomy appears to increase oxygenation of the macula. Kadonoso and colleagues [14] demonstrated increased perifoveal capillary blood flow after vitrectomy in their series. Stefansson and associates [15,16] reported that vitrectomy with lensectomy allows aqueous to provide increased levels of oxygen to the inner retina and that movement of oxygen transcorneally to the vitreous has been demonstrated to be more effective in vitrectomized eyes [17]. Therefore, vitrectomy has been reported to be beneficial in these situations. Some studies, however, have shown that vitrectomy is effective even when there is no evidence of macular traction [18-21]. Perhaps this is due to removal of the posterior hyaloid also removes toxic substances, such as histamine, free radical scavengers, and VEGF, which may be harbored in the preretinal space [22].

Recent advances in vitreous surgery have enabled us to treat surgically eyes with good visual acuity. The critical process in vitrectomy is making complete posterior vitreous detachment and removing the thickened and attached posterior hyaloids. We have used multifocal electroretinogram technique to investigate the effects of vitrectomy on macular visual function for diabetic ME, and prospectively evaluated the surgical outcomes in visual function. It's concluded that vitrectomy is helpful not only in reducing ME, and improving best correct visual acuity, but also in reinforcing the resume of macular and paramacular visual function [23]. (Fig. 2)

3. Vitrectomy with ILM peel

Recently, ILM peeling has been added to the procedure of surgical treatment for ME. Addition of ILM peel to vitrectomy expedites the resolution of the ME and prevents its recurrence, which would appear to enhance the beneficial effects of vitrectomy [24]. The mechanism for this was postulated to be the elimination of all tractional forces at the vitreoretinal interface and removal of the scaffold used by astrocytes to proliferate on the retinal surface. In additon, it was hypothesized that vitrectomy with removal of the ILM would allow the ME to decompress by facilitating the release of extracellular fluid into the vitreous, which would, in turn, restore normal retinal thickness and intraretinal tissue pressure. Challenges in surgical manipulation include poor visibility of the thin transparent membrane and the small dimensions and the sensitivity of the macular tissue. More recently, many study demonstrated that the technical difficulty of performing ILM peels can be eased with staining that specifically targets the ILM [25-29], which including indocyanine green, triamcinolone acetonide, trypan blue, whole blood, and brilliant blue G. These were shown selectively to stain the ILM and not the posterior vitreous or the underlying retinal layers. The use of indocyanine green in ILM removal has been decreased more recently for several reports of indocyanine green toxicity. Triamcinolone acetonide, trypan blue and brilliant blue G have become popularly used in ILM staining. (Fig. 3) We have treated chronic cystoid ME in branch retinal vein occlusion with 25-gauge vitrectomy and TA-assisted ILM peeling, and evaluated the efficacy. The result is that TA-assisted ILM peeling is generally effective in reducing ME and improving BCVA for CCME in BRVO for at least 7 months [30]. Certainly, the ILM can also be peeled without a visualization agent to avoid concerns of toxicity, especially if the ocular media and surgeon's view are particularly clear. This would avoid dye toxicity concerns but runs the risk of incomplete peeling. But in cases of ME, the adhesion of the ILM to the macula is stronger, and the manipulation must be more delicate. Therefore, additional repeated staining may be indicated, which decrease the risk of iatrogenic damage from surgical manipulation. Nevertheless, the value of ILM removal for treatment of ME has also been questioned recently. In a study of 135 eyes, 74 of which underwent ILM peeling, Kumagai and associates [31] found that even though ILM removal accelerated the absorption of ME, the final VA and rate of ME absorption were similar in both groups.

4. Vitrectomy with intravitreous pharmacologic therapies

Recently, intravitreous pharmacologic therapies (including intravitreal TA, VEGF inhibitors and protein kinase C beta-isoform inhibitors) have been demonstrated as effective in the treatment of ME when other modalities have failed, especially laser, in the setting of retinal vascular decompensation ME [32-34]. Intravitreous corticosteroids such as TA have been documented to reduce macular leakage in ME retinopathy with or without clinically

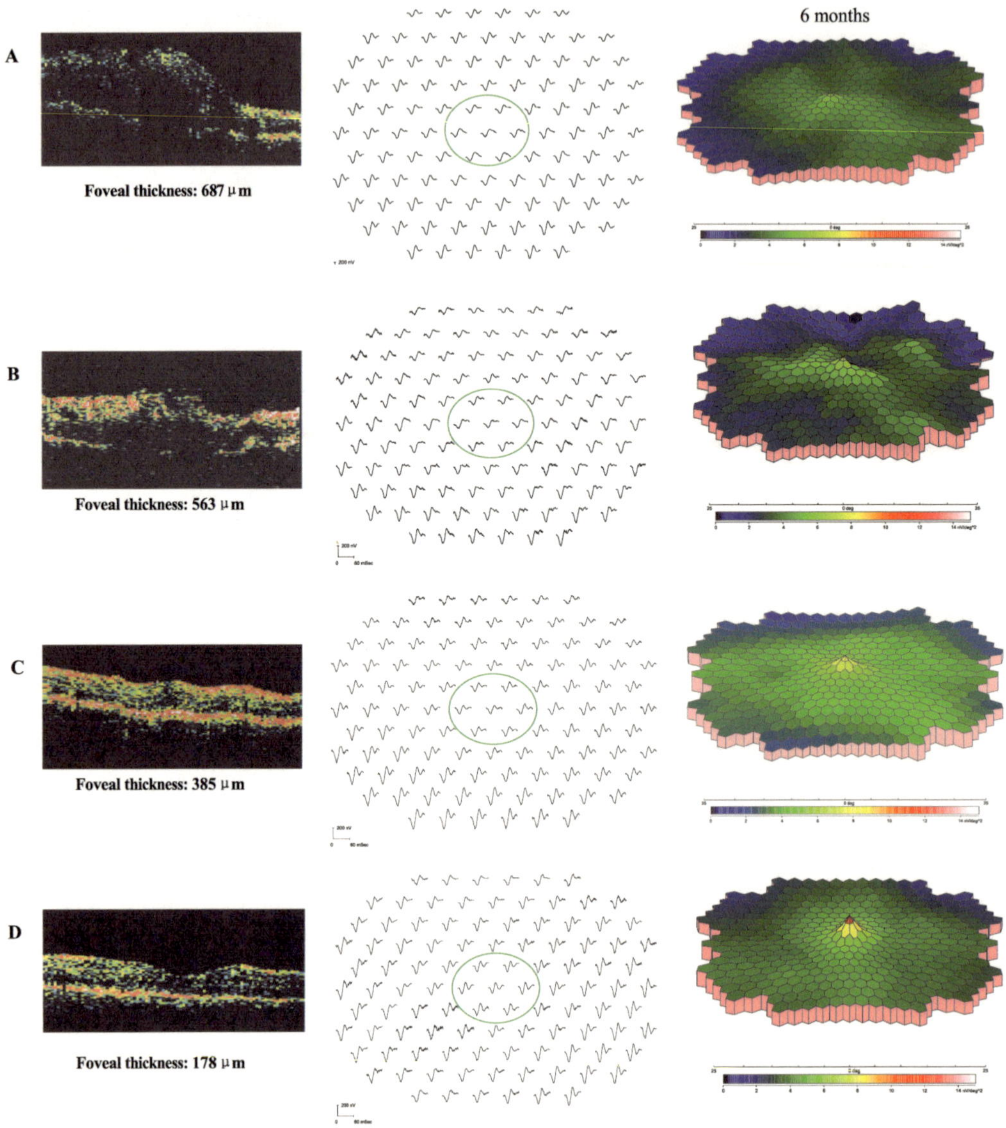

(A) before vitrectomy, the P1 value of amplitude and latency were 5.8 nv/deg² and 41.6 msec respectively; the best-corrected visual acuity was 0.04. (B) 2 months after vitrectomy, the P1 value of amplitude and latency were 6.3 nv/deg² and 40.2 msec respectively; the best-corrected visual acuity was 0.08. (C) 4 months after vitrectomy, the P1 value of amplitude and latency were 11.4 nv/deg² and 32.7 msec respectively; the best-corrected visual acuity was 0.2. (D) 6 months after vitrectomy, the P1 value of amplitude and latency were 16.9 nv/deg² and 25.3 msec respectively; the best-corrected visual acuity was 0.3. Ovals indicate central hexagons (ring1 and ring2 area). (From Ma J et al. Assessment of Macular Function by Multifocal Electroretinogram in Diabetic Macular Edema before and after Vitrectomy. Documenta Ophthalmologica. 2004;109 (2): 131-137.)

Fig. 2. The OCT image (left), trace array (Middle) and 3-D topography (right) of multifocal ERG for a same case of diabetic macular edema. With the passage of follow up, macular edema had decreased and retinal fuction had increased gradually.

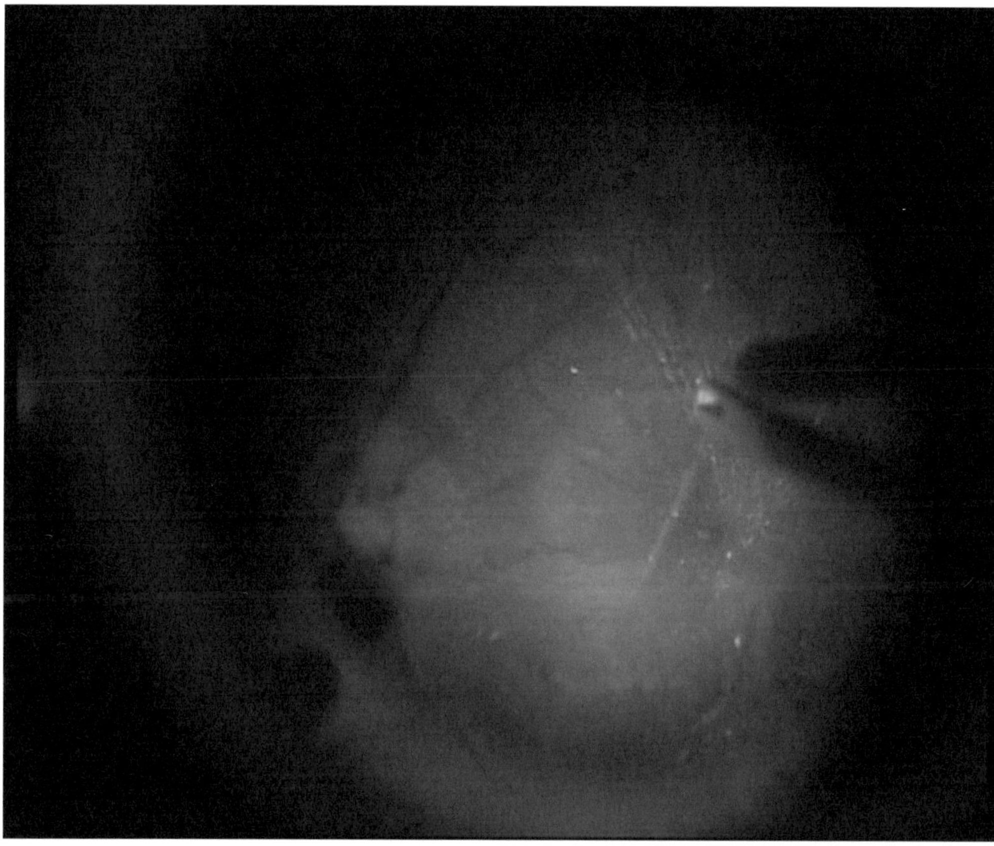

Fig. 3. Triamcinolone acetonide (TA) assisted internal limiting membrane (ILM)-peeling. The ILM is directly grasped with an intraocular forceps and peeled in a circumferential manner around the macular edema. The peeled area is clearly observed as lacking the whites specks left by the TA. (Supplied by Jin Ma, MD.)

significant traction from vitreous or preretinal membranes. In this setting, corticosteroids appear to be effective by inhibiting both VEGF and macrophage-released factors on the basis of mechanisms described here. Corticosteroids may also be important in promoting overall endothelial cell repair [35]. VEGF is a peptide growth factor specific for vascular endothelial cells and increases vascular permeability and is thought to contribute to capillary wall dysfunction [36]. VEGF plays a dominant role in retinal vascular leakage and formation of ME. VEGF-A has been implicated as an important factor in the breakdown of the blood–retina barrier, with increased vascular permeability resulting in retinal edema in diabetes by affecting endothelial tight junction proteins [37]. Therefore, VEGF inhibition is another promising pharmacologic approach in the management of ME. There are several different anti-VEGF drugs which have been used in the management of ME, including pegaptanib (Macugen; Eyetech Pharmaceuticals, New York, New York, USA), bevacizumab (Avastin; Genentech Inc.), and ranibizumab (Lucentis; Genentech Inc., South San Francisco, California). Ruboxistaurin, a selective protein kinase C binhibitor, reduced retinal vascular leakage in patients with diabetic ME and reduced the rate of sustained moderate visual loss in those with moderately severe to very severe non proliferative diabetic retinopathy [32].

During the surgery, intravitreous pharmaceuticals mentioned above should be drop on the surface of fovea, after surgical removal of the posterior hyaloids with or without ILM peeling, and an air–fluid exchange carried out. Thus, vitrectomy with intravitreous pharmacologic combined therapies could provide clinicians with a set of power tools to treat ME, and may lead to a synergistic benefit that is not observed with monotherapy.

5. Removal of hard exudates and cysts

Further surgical procedures for ME are being attempted. Longstanding macular deposits may cause macular dysfunction and macular atrophy [38]. Direct removal of hard exudates was attempted by Takagi et al. [39] in a series of 7 eyes with massive hard exudates. They performed removal of the exudates by aspiration with a silicone-tipped extrusion needle or by direct removal with intraocular forceps. The final postoperative visual acuity was bad. In addition, intraoperative iatrogenic macular holes can be caused by the removal of neural retina surrounding the removed exudates. This complication rate mandates caution in using this technique.

Tachi et al. [40] attempted treatment of diabetic cystoid ME with cystotomy or cystectomy in addition to vitrectomy with posterior hyaloid removal. Despite resolution of cystoid ME in a few cases, there were several reported complications, including intraoperative retinal tears, and cyst reformation. The study could not demonstrate that this technique was superior to vitrectomy and posterior hyaloid removal alone.

6. Conclusions

Even so, laser photocoagulation remains the treatment of choice for ME associated with nondiffuse patterns of vascular leakage [41]. The action of photocoagulation is not fully known, but it is suspected that the method of treatment as described here not only cauterizes focally leaking sites, but also leads to vasoconstriction, the latter possibly by decreasing oxygen consumption in the outer retinal layers and increasing oxygen tension in the inner retinal layers [42]. Vitreous surgery is often effective in resolving ME associated with vitreoretinal or epiretinal traction and yields variable results in nontractional cases. A variety of pharmacologic agents targeting inflammatory and vasopermeability molecules have been shown to reduce diffuse ME and improve visual function over the short-term. Although treatment options continue to expand with the development of new drugs and surgical procedures, the long-term efficacy and safety of most new approaches have yet to be established in randomized, controlled clinical trials. We should be clear that this is a complicated disease which has been far than thoroughly investigated, which needs our further research on its pathogenesis thus leading to the introduction of additional pharmacological agents for the treatment and reduction of visual loss of ME. A variety of promising new medical and surgical therapies are under investigation, but additional clinical research is required to determine their role alone or in combination.

7. References

[1] Enden MK, Nyengaard JR, Ostrow E, et al. Elevated glucose levels increase retinal glycolysis and sorbitol pathway metabolism. *Invest Ophthalmol Vis Sci.* 1994;53:2968–2975.

[2] Kristinsson JK, Gottfendsdottir MS, Stefansson E. Retinal vessel dilatation and elongation precedes diabetic macular edema. *Br J Opthalmol.* 1997;81:274–278.

[3] Parving HH, Vibenti GC, Kern H, et al. Hemodynamic factors in the genesis of diabetic microangiopathy. *Metabolism*. 1983;32:993-999.
[4] Abbasi M, Covantoni M, Chu L, et al. Adhesiveness of mononuclear cells to endothelium in patients with NIDDM. *Diabetes*. 1996;45(suppl):66.
[5] Yoshida A, Feke GT, Morales-Stoppello J. et al. Retinal blood flow alterations during progression of diabetic retinopathy. *Arch Ophthalmol*. 1983;101:225-227.
[6] Sebag J, Buckingham B, Charles MA, et al. Biochemical abnormalities in vitreous of humans with proliferative diabetic retinopathy. *Arch Ophthalmol*. 1992;110:1472-1476.
[7] Sebag J, Boulazs EA. Pathogenesis of CME: Anatomic considerations of vitreoretinal adhesion. *Surv Ophthalmol*. 1984;29(suppl):493-498.
[8] Sebag J. Diabetic vitreopathy. Ophthalmology. 1996;103:205-206.
[9] Jumper MJ, Embabi SN, Toth CA, et al. Electron immunocytochemical analysis of protein hyaloid associated with diabetic macular edema. Retina. 2000;20:63-68.
[10] Lewis H. The role of vitrectomy in the treatment of diabetic macular edema. Am J Ophthalmol. 2001;131:123-125.
[11] Schepens CL, Avila MP, Jalkh AE, et al. Role of the vitreous in cystoid;macular edema. Surv Ophthalmol. 1984;28(suppl):499-504.
[12] Nasrallah FP, Van de Velde F, Jalkh AE, et allL. Importance of the vitreous in young diabetics with macular edema. Ophthalmology. 1989;96:1511-1517.
[13] Massin P, Duguid G, Erginay A, et al. Optical coherence tomography for evaluating diabetic macular edema before and after vitrectomy. Am J Ophthalmol. 2003;135:169-177.
[14] Kadonosono K, Itoh N, Ohno S. Perifoveal microcirculation before and after vitrectomy for diabetic cystoid macular edema. Am J Ophthalmol. 2000;130:740-744.
[15] Stefansson E, Landers MB 3rd, Wobarsht ML. Increased retinal oxygen supply following panretinal photocoagulation and vitrectomy and lensectomy. Trans Am Ophthal Soc. 1981;79:307-334.
[16] Stefansson E. The therapeutic effects of retinal laser treatment and vitrectomy. A theory based on oxygen and vascular physiology. Acta Ophthalmol Scand. 2001;79:435-440.
[17] Wilson CA, Benner JD, Berkowitz BA, et al. Transcorneal oxygenation of the preretinal vitreous. Arch Ophthalmol. 1994;112:839-845.
[18] Tachi N, Ogino N. Vitrectomy for diffuse macular edema in cases of diabetic retinopathy. Am J Ophthalmol 1996; 122:258-260.
[19] La Heij EC, Hendrikse F, Kessels AGH, Derhaag PJFM. Vitrectomy results in diabetic macular edema without evident vitreomacular traction. Graefes Arch Clin Exp Ophthalmol 2001; 239:264-270.
[20] Yanyali A, Horozoglu F, Celik E, Nohutcu AF. Long-term outcomes of pars plana vitrectomy with internal limiting membrane removal in diabetic macular edema. Retina 2007; 27:557-566.
[21] Patel JI, Hykin PG, Schadt M, et al. Pars plana vitrectomy for diabetic macular oedema: OCT and functional correlations. Eye 2006; 20:674-680.
[22] Christoforidis JB, D'Amico DJ. Surgical and other treatments of diabetic macular edema: an update.Int Ophthalmol Clin. 2004 ;44(1):139-60.
[23] Ma J, Yao K, Jiang J, Wu D, Gao R, Yin J, Fang X. Assessment of macular function by multifocal electroretinogram in diabetic macular edema before and after vitrectomy. Doc Ophthalmol. 2004;109(2):131-7.
[24] Gandorfer A, Messmer EM, Ulbig MW, et al. Resolution of diabetic macular edema after surgical removal of the posterior hyaloid and the inner limiting membrane. Retina. 2000;20:126-133.

[25] Mochizuki Y, Enaida H, Hisatomi T, Hata Y, Miura M, Arita R, Kawahara S, Kita T, Ueno A, Ishibashi T. The internal limiting membrane peeling with brilliant blue G staining for retinal detachment due to macular hole in high myopia. Br J Ophthalmol. 2008;92(7):1009.
[26] Oie Y, Emi K, Takaoka G, Ikeda T. Effect of indocyanine green staining in peeling of internal limiting membrane for retinal detachment resulting from macular hole in myopic eyes. Ophthalmology. 2007;114(2):303-6.
[27] Lai CC, Wu WC, Chuang LH, Yeung L, Lee JS, Chen TL. Selective staining of the internal limiting membrane using the sequential intraoperative instillation of whole blood followed by indocyanine green dye. Am J Ophthalmol. 2005;140(2):320-2.
[28] Azad RV, Pal N, Vashisht N, Sharma YR, Kumar A. Efficacy of 0.15% trypan blue for staining and removal of the internal limiting membrane, epiretinal membranes, and the posterior hyaloid during pars plana vitrectomy. Retina. 2005;25(5):676.
[29] Tognetto D, Zenoni S, Sanguinetti G, Haritoglou C, Ravalico G. Staining of the internal limiting membrane with intravitreal triamcinolone acetonide. Retina. 2005; 25(4):462-7.
[30] Ma J, Yao K, Zhang Z, Tang X. 25-gauge vitrectomy and triamcinolone acetonide-assisted internal limiting membrane peeling for chronic cystoid macular edema associated with branch retinal vein occlusion. Retina. 2008;28(7):947-56.
[31] Kumagai K, Ogino N, Furukawa M, et al. Internal limiting membrane peeling in vitreous surgery for diabetic macular edema. Nippon Ganka Gakkai Zasshi. 2002;106:590–594.
[32] Frank RN. Potential new medical therapies for diabetic retinopathy: Protein kinase C inhibitors. Am J Ophthalmol. 2002;133:693–698.
[33] Haritoglou C, Kook D, Neubauer A, et al. Intravitreal bevacizumab (Avastin) therapy for persistent diffuse diabetic macular edema. Retina 2006; 26:999–1005.
[34] Gillies MC, Sutter FK, Simpson JM, et al. Intravitreal triamcinolone for refractory diabetic macular edema: two-year results of a double-masked, placebocontrolled, randomized clinical trial. Ophthalmology 2006; 113:1533–1538.
[35] Gibran SK, Khan K, Jungkim S, Cleary PE. Optical coherence tomographic pattern may predict visual outcome after intravitreal triamcinolone for diabetic macular edema. Ophthalmology 2007; 114:890–894.
[36] Vinores SA, Youssri AI, Luna JD, et al. Upregulation of vascular endothelial growth factor in ischemic and non-ischemic human and experimental retinal disease. Histol Histopathol. 1997;12:99–109.
[37] Qaum T, Xu Q, Joussen AM, et al. VEGF-initiated blood-retinal barrier breakdown in early diabetes. Invest Ophthalmol Vis Sci 2001; 42:2408–2413.
[38] Davis MD, Fisher MR, Gangnon RE, et al. Risk factors for high-risk proliferative diabetic retinopathy and severe visual loss: Early Treatment Diabetic Retinopathy Study. Report #18. Invest Ophthalmol Vis Sci. 1998;39:233–252.
[39] Takagi H, Otani A, Kiryu J, et al. New surgical approach for removing massive foveal hard exudates in diabetic macular edema. Ophthalmology. 1999;106:249–256.
[40] Tachi N, Hashimoto Y, Ogino N. Cystotomy for diabetic cystoid macular edema. Doc Ophthalmol. 1999;97(3–4):459–463.
[41] Johnson MW. Etiology and treatment of macular edema. Am J Ophthalmol. 2009; 147(1):11-21.
[42] Weiter JJ, Zuckerman R. The influence of the photoreceptor RPE complex on the inner retina. Ophthalmology. 1980;87:1133–1139.